Worry-Free Dentistry
At Last!

DR. SCOTT BILLINGS & DR. CHRISTOPHER MURPHY

Worry-Free Dentistry
At Last!

A PATIENT'S GUIDE TO ANXIETY-FREE DENTISTRY

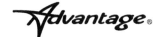

Published by Advantage, Charleston, South Carolina.
Member of Advantage Media Group.

ADVANTAGE is a registered trademark, and the Advantage colophon is a trademark of Advantage Media Group, Inc.

Printed in the United States of America.

10 9 8 7 6 5 4 3 2 1

ISBN: 978-1-59932-958-1

Book design by Carly Blake.

This publication is designed to provide accurate and authoritative information in regard to the subject matter covered. It is sold with the understanding that the publisher is not engaged in rendering legal, accounting, or other professional services. If legal advice or other expert assistance is required, the services of a competent professional person should be sought.

Advantage Media Group is proud to be a part of the Tree Neutral® program. Tree Neutral offsets the number of trees consumed in the production and printing of this book by taking proactive steps such as planting trees in direct proportion to the number of trees used to print books. To learn more about Tree Neutral, please visit www.treeneutral.com.

Advantage Media Group is a publisher of business, self-improvement, and professional development books and online learning. We help entrepreneurs, business leaders, and professionals share their Stories, Passion, and Knowledge to help others Learn & Grow. Do you have a manuscript or book idea that you would like us to consider for publishing? Please visit advantagefamily.com or call 1.866.775.1696.

Dr. Scott Billings

I wish to dedicate this book to my wife, Debbie. When you've been together for forty-two years, you become a team. Debbie is so often able to help me view things with a perspective that I'm not able to see on my own. I always value her advice and the comfort she gives when I have challenges in front of me.

Dr. Chris Murphy

I am dedicating this book to my wife and life partner Laura. At an age when most dentists are either winding down or retiring, Dr. Billings and I have decided to continue our dedication to our patients. I am very grateful that I have a wonderful wife who sees that and is so supportive and understanding.

We also want to dedicate this book to the team at Eastern Shore Dental Care. You have helped thousands of patients who have been anxious about going to the dentist. Your compassion and care has helped change their lives.

Table of Contents

Introduction

If you're reading this, the chances are that you suffer from some degree of dental anxiety or phobia—a fear of visiting a dentist or of having your teeth worked on. If that's your situation, know that you're not alone; about 75 percent of Americans suffer from some degree of dental anxiety, according to research quoted in *The Journal of the American Dental Association*,[1] while another study, published in *The Journal of Dental Hygiene*, revealed that more than 20 percent of dentally anxious patients do not see a dentist regularly, and anywhere from 9 to 15 percent of anxious patients avoid care altogether.[2]

Unfortunately, because they're not getting the treatment they need, their teeth may hurt every time they eat. When they talk to people, they're likely to use their hands to hide their mouths, because of embarrassment over missing or discolored teeth. Those who avoid regular dental exams and treatment can also expect to have increased incidence of gum disease which, left unchecked, can have serious

---

1   R.A. Kleinknecht et al., "Factor Analysis of the Dental Fear Survey with Cross-Validation," *J Am Dent Assoc.* 108, no. 1(January 1984): 59-61, https://www.ncbi.nlm.nih.gov/pubmed/6582116.

2   Angela M. White, Lori Giblin, and Linda D. Boyd, "The Prevalence of Dental Anxiety in Dental Practice Settings," American Dental Hygienists' Association 91, no. 1 (February 2017): 30-34, https://www.ncbi.nlm.nih.gov/pubmed/29118148.

consequences for their overall health. When pain finally forces them to go to the dentist, their treatment needs are likely to be extensive—and that makes them even more fearful. Very often, instead of receiving the treatment they need to get them back to good dental health, they will only get enough treatment to stop the pain and then continue to avoid the dentist.

Does any of this sound familiar? If so, there's something we want you to know: there is hope—and help—for you. Dental anxiety is a terrible thing, but we know that you can't help feeling the way you do. You wish you didn't, you're embarrassed by it, and you'd give anything not to have these fears—but you do, and you feel overwhelmed by them. While you may never wholly conquer your fears, a caring practitioner can help you to get the care you need with minimal discomfort or anxiety, and you deserve no less.

So many dentists just don't get it; whether it's because they're simply not empathic people, or because they're so sure that they're not going to hurt the patient that they rush people and push them outside of their comfort zones. How many times has a dentist told you, "This isn't going to hurt"—and then subsequently hurt you? How many times have your fears been dismissed or shrugged off when you've been brave enough to share your feelings, with, "Oh, come on now, you're an adult, not a little kid—you should know better"? Maybe the worst is when your pain anesthetic hasn't worked the way it's supposed to, and the dentist keeps telling you, "You can't be feeling that!" when you know you are.

If it's happened to you as it has to so many people, then you know that's no comfort at all. We've been the doctors, but we've also been the patients in the chair—and we've had those kinds of experiences, too. That's not the kind of practice we want to go to, much less to have ourselves.

We've been in practice together since 1986, and we've been very successful at helping even our most fearful patients feel comfortable in the dentist's chair. Everything about our offices, down to the colors on the wall and the chairs themselves, is designed to make you relax and feel safe. But the most important thing about the way we work is how we treat you—with respect, sensitivity, and patience. We don't try to talk you out of your feelings, we don't talk down to you, and we don't dismiss your fears; we listen. Once we know

> We put the power back in your hands. To put it simply— we understand.

what your issues are, then together we come up with strategies to work around them so that you can get the care you need. We go slow, if that's what you prefer. We put the power back in your hands. To put it simply—we understand.

Our mission is your health; our passion is compassionate care. They don't teach that skill set in dental school, although they should. Over the years, we've expanded the scope of the accommodations and comforts we offer our fearful patients, and the many, many referrals we've had from both dentists and patients are a great testimony to our success. We're here to help you, not judge you—because we know that these fears that afflict you aren't your fault.

Dental phobias most often spring from having had a bad experience at the hands of an uncaring or insensitive practitioner during childhood, though fears can also be "inherited," in the sense that a parent who suffers with them can pass those fears along to their child. And as anyone who suffers from them can tell you, it's not "all in their head." Phobias can cause intense physical and emotional reactions. Some people may not be able to sleep the night before they go to the dentist; others may feel physically ill at the thought of it. Some patients begin to feel anxious as they enter the waiting room. Sweaty palms, a rapid heart rate, and confusion are common. For those most powerfully affected, their reactions can be much more severe, and they may start to panic or gag when the dentist begins to place his or her hands in their mouths. As practitioners who focus on working with anxious patients, we have had many instances where we've entered a room to meet a patient seated in the dental chair, only to have the patient burst into uncontrollable tears at the sight of us. Some people are so phobic that they can't even enter the treatment room.

But the good news is that we've been able to help many people, including those who had previously found it impossible to get treatment. We've restored missing teeth, ended years of discomfort, and brought smiles back to the faces of hundreds of patients, and seeing their happiness and relief is the most rewarding part of our work. One of our patients tells us every time she comes in, "Promise me you won't ever retire!" This is a woman who literally couldn't bring herself to sit in the dental chair when she first came to us. It took time and patience, but now she is getting to her regularly scheduled exams and cleanings with no anxiety at all, and she couldn't be prouder of her new appearance.

In this book, we'll be examining all aspects of dental phobias— where they come from, the many ways in which they can manifest themselves, and how a caring and compassionate dentist can help you get past them. We'll empower you with information and help you to learn how to ask for and get what you need, in terms of accommodations. We'll put the power to get the care you need back into your hands.

Since there are two of us, we have each written alternating chapters, each sharing our own stories and those of our patients with you. We hope in the course of this book to answer all your questions, to help you take the first steps to reclaiming your oral health, and to assist you in getting that beautiful smile you've been missing.

CHAPTER 1

What Is Dental Phobia?

Dr. Chris Murphy

I t is so often the first question we're asked by a new patient that I've lost count of how many times I've heard it: "Am I the worst patient you've ever had?"

The answer is always the same—"No way, you're not even in the top one thousand!" Our practice brings us into contact with so many fearful patients that there's very little, if anything, we haven't seen and dealt with in terms of helping people through their treatment. And there are numerous levels of fearfulness and multiple triggers that provoke them. Some people can overcome these fears with minimal assistance, but others need more help.

For one person, it might be a fear of needles that is particularly acute at the dentist's office. For another, the fear might be associated with claustrophobia (the fear of narrow or enclosed spaces) that is exacerbated by reclining in the dental chair with people, instruments, and machinery hovering over them. For others, it's the sense of their own vulnerability, or the sound of the drill or other machinery that triggers anxiety. The good news is that it's possible to get past fears and gradually overcome them—with the support of an understanding dentist.

> What are the feelings that overwhelm you when you consider a visit to the dentist?

What are the feelings that overwhelm you when you consider a visit to the dentist? Is it loss of control? Fear of the instruments, the smells of dental chemicals, fear of the dentist or hygienist? Is it fear of pain?

THE MOST COMMON FEARS

Fear of being judged for poor oral health or appearance

Chances are that if you have dental fear or dental phobia, you avoid the dentist as much as you possibly can. Obviously, that's not going to be good for your oral health, and may mean that your teeth are in rough shape when you finally do come in. I can tell you that no matter how damaged your teeth are, *we will not judge you*. We're here to bring you back to health and to restore your appearance. The bigger the challenge that restorative work presents, the bigger the improvement will be. And we're well aware that coming in at all required a real effort on your part. We're glad you're here, and we'll do our best to make it as easy as possible.

Fear of being powerless

This is a very common issue for people who fear dental work, and it's easy to see why. Most of the time when you go into the dentist's offices, you're whisked from the waiting room to the treatment room and into a chair. Nobody who works there thinks of taking a few minutes to talk with you, to see how you're feeling and ask you if you need anything to make your experience more comfortable. You're put in a vulnerable-feeling supine position, with peoples' hands and instruments in your mouth. Nobody's telling you what's happening or what they're doing; if they're talking at all, it's to each other. Feeling powerless is particularly terrifying for those who have been abused as children; they may literally be unable to stand the stress reaction it creates.

Our philosophy is to give the power back to the patient, and we start by making it clear that we can and will stop, for as long as you need, if you just raise your hand. We're also alert for other signs that you may be feeling overwhelmed and will stop immediately to check in with you. For the record, I had a run-in as a kid with a dentist who was in such a hurry to get through my procedure that he proceeded even when I told him that it hurt. He'd started out well enough, telling me that if I felt pain, I should hold up my hand and he'd stop and numb me up a little more. And that worked, the first two or three times—then he got impatient. "Just hold still," he snapped, "We'll be done in a minute!" and he continued to drill. I remember very clearly thinking, "Man, I wish you were the person in the chair, and I was the one with the drill—we'd see how long a minute feels to you!"

Fear of being hurt

This makes perfect sense to anyone who's ever been hurt by a dentist—especially when they're telling you that you "should" be numb, or you "can't possibly" be feeling any pain. In fact, the chemicals your body releases during a stress reaction makes it harder for painkilling drugs to take effect, and if you suffer from dental fear or phobia, then that's a good indicator that you may need a higher dose of those medications than does a person who does not have fear. We don't move forward at all until we're sure you're numb.

And if on a given day we just can't numb you sufficiently to get you through a procedure, then we send you home. We never proceed when a patient tells us they're uncomfortable, and we never try to shame them or insist they're not feeling what they clearly are feeling. That's disrespectful and insensitive.

Fear of gagging or choking

This one's another very common fear, and it's especially uncomfortable for these people to have impressions taken with the dreaded "tray of goop." For some folks with an overactive gag reflex, this is very unpleasant because they're afraid they'll vomit during a procedure. And that does occasionally happen, but it's not a big deal and nothing you should be ashamed about. Fortunately, most impressions can be done virtually now with a 3-D scanner. Interestingly, there are simple exercises you can do to lessen your gag reflex. One is to take a wooden tongue depressor and rest it on your tongue, gradually moving it back toward your throat until the reflex kicks in. Rest a moment, then try again. Work on getting it back a little further every night until you can feel the reflex lessening. While you may not entirely cure your gag reflex this way, you can certainly improve it and make it less of a worry to you.

Fear of not being able to breathe

This is a very common fear, and again, perfectly understandable, given that during dental work hands and instruments are around and in your mouth. We find that periodic and frequent pauses in treatment are very helpful, and that, again, putting the power in the patient's hands to stop the treatment at any moment really helps to tamp down this fear.

Fear of lying down in the dental chair and being placed in a vulnerable position

This is a common one, and often springs from sometimes-undiagnosed claustrophobia. Sometimes it's an after-effect of having been sexually abused in childhood, even if the memory of the abuse itself has been buried. When we have a patient with this fear, we work on them with the chair in a fully upright position. That's more difficult for us, but it makes it possible for the patient to get through their procedure with significantly less stress, and that's a win for everyone.

> We find that noise-cancelling headphones work wonders for those people who can't stand the sound of the drill.

Fear of the drill

There's a lot to dislike about the dental drill. Some people find the noise it makes alarming; for many, it's the memory of pain it has inflicted, when they weren't adequately numbed up by a previous dentist. We find that noise-cancelling headphones work wonders for those people who can't stand the sound of the drill, and that, again, being responsive and quick to stop significantly helps those who fear pain.

Fear of having the jaw lock up

Having your mouth open for more than a few minutes at a time can be very uncomfortable, and some patients are worried that it won't close properly. This won't happen unless you have a very specific TMJ issue, and hopefully we'd know about that ahead of time. If the jaw should lock up, the dentist's office is probably the best place to be—but it's rare, and again, would be connected to a specific issue with the jaw. If you do have jaw issues, discuss them with your dentist. We find that, for a lot of these people, using dental bite blocks lessens the stress of holding the mouth open.

Fear of being victimized or abused

This is an awful one, and so hard for people who have been victims of abuse to cope with. While this is most often tied to childhood abuse by a trusted adult, I have run into a few patients in my career who were physically or verbally abused by dentists, and I can't imagine how much courage it took them to get them into a dentist's office again after an experience like that. Other times, people have been frightened in the past by a dentist who was verbally abusive to either the patient or the staff, shouting and throwing instruments down during a procedure. That's appalling behavior and completely unprofessional, and certainly not something you'll ever see here. Please be as open with your dentist as you can about what accommodations you need to feel safe. You don't have to tell them about your personal history if you're not comfortable with doing that, but please do ask for what you need. If that means you require frequent breaks, comfort objects, having someone hold your hand during your procedure, or having your spouse in the room, that's fine.

Fear of blood

Many people get weak or even faint at the sight of blood, and some procedures do entail a little bleeding—even a cleaning, particularly if the person hasn't been taking care of their teeth and there's some gum disease that's causing inflammation. But we can help you get past that by making sure you don't see it.

Fear of being closed in, or claustrophobia

While this is a really uncomfortable and even terrifying feeling for those who suffer from it, it's one of the things with which we're able to easily help patients to cope, just by making some special modifications. Frequent breaks during treatment so that the patient can sit up unencumbered help a lot. And we've designed our offices to have high ceilings, too, to lessen that closed in feeling.

Fear of having your personal space encroached on

Sometimes this is a cultural thing, but most often it's a form of claustrophobia or connected with past abuse. Again, the most effective way to deal with it is to let the patient dictate the terms of treatment, and by letting them take a break whenever they need it and for as long as they need it. Some people prefer to have a lot of short appointments because they can't deal with longer ones, and that's fine too.

There are many levels and kinds of anxiety that patients can manifest. For instance, we had a patient who had a consuming fear that somehow, when we did nearly anything to her teeth—even a cleaning—it would make them fall out. For that patient, a discussion about the procedure, showing her what we are doing in a mirror, and explaining that her teeth are strongly engaged in her jaw and that they will not come out, was all it took to relieve her fears. But somehow, she'd never come across a dentist who was willing to listen or to make that small effort to reassure her.

Another patient I worked with was deathly afraid of getting injections. Validating her concerns, and letting her know that we understand that many people feel that way, but that we a way to give injections comfortably, allowed her to get her treatment done.

Then there are the patients that have more extreme reactions to being in the office at all. For those patients, we can see that they are visibly shaken at the onset of their appointment. Our staff members (who are trained here to spot signs of distress when they talk with our patients) meet them first, and will let us know that the patient is extremely anxious, so that we are prepared to walk into the room and help them with their fears. Sometimes when they see us for the first time, they begin to sob uncontrollably even before we exchange words. This type of patient needs extra special care for them to be able to be helped by us—care we're willing and able to provide.

> As a patient, you deserve to be treated compassionately and with respect, not rushed, not dismissed, and not forced beyond the limits of your comfort zone.

With any kind of fear or phobia, the keys for getting past it and getting patients the care they need are patience and validation of patients' feelings. As a patient, you deserve to be treated compassionately and with respect, not rushed, not dismissed, and not forced beyond the limits of your comfort zone. Any dentist should be willing to respect those boundaries and give you what you need to feel comfortable. If your dentist isn't willing to do this, then it's time to try another dentist.

CHAPTER 2

The Origins of Dental Anxiety and Phobias

Dr. Scott Billings

Where do the fears and phobias that keep people away from the dentist begin? The answer to that is as varied as the human experience, but very often we find that it begins in childhood, with a bad experience that leaves a lifelong mark on the patient.

Sometimes, the problem stems from rough or frightening treatment they got from a dentist. It used to be quite common when working on children to use what's called a "papoose board," which is a restraining device that effectively straps the child into place so that they can't wiggle or move during treatment. Thank heaven, these are going out of fashion among enlightened practitioners (and if you have children, please don't ever allow these devices to be used on them!), because being forcibly immobilized can be a traumatizing experience that leaves a patient with a lifetime fear and distrust of dentists generally, and it's easy to see why.

Sometimes, parents are asked to restrain a child and hold them down in the chair, which can also be a terrible experience for a frightened child, especially since the parent is now in league with their tormentor, as the child sees it.

We've talked about how sexual or other physical abuse can leave psychological scars that can be triggered by a trip to the dentist; if you or a member of your family has had these kinds of experiences, I hope that you can find the courage to seek professional help and healing. And while you're certainly not obliged to share this with your dentist, please do tell him or her what procedures or postures make you anxious, so they know to avoid them.

WHEN DENTISTS AREN'T SUITED TO THEIR PROFESSION

The vast majority of dentists are thoughtful, caring professionals—but not all of them. Technical skills can only take a practitioner so far. A dentist also needs people skills—empathy, tact, and humor are all helpful—because without those, even a skilled technician isn't really a good match for the profession. And some are even less emotionally suited to our work than that: short-tempered, snappish, or even rough, usually because they're in a hurry to move on to another patient.

> The vast majority of dentists are thoughtful, caring professionals—but not all of them.

And yes, there is probably a minute group that enjoys their patients' discomfort. But most of the time, they just aren't being careful enough, or caring enough.

If you've suffered at the hands of a *Little Shop of Horrors*-style dentist who inflicted pain, it's only natural that you're going to be distrustful going forward, and that can translate to phobia. For example, we often get patients who are afraid of getting painkilling shots in their mouths because the experience has been so painful in the past. For one of my patients, Carly, this was especially problematic.

I was working on Carly one day when we were doing a crown procedure; part of that procedure requires squirting impression material on a tooth with a syringe that looks a lot like a needle. When the assistant put the syringe in my hand—and before I had a chance to tell Carly what it really was—poor Carly whipped her head away so quickly she nearly hurt us both. She was that terrified of needles, because of having had a dentist who had given her an injection as a kid without preparing her or warning her that she was would feel some pain. After that experience, she just didn't trust dentists. In this situation, I had talked her through getting a shot so that we were able to numb her for the procedure, and we prepared the tooth. But even after all that, when I came at her with something when she wasn't forewarned, she responded violently.

People who have been hurt by dentists find it tough to trust dentists, and that's especially true if it happened in childhood. I've had patients of very advanced years who could describe to me in detail the traumatic experience they had when they were eight or ten years old, at the hands of an impatient or unskilled practitioner.

> People who have been hurt by dentists find it tough to trust dentists, and that's especially true if it happened in childhood.

THE ISSUES OF PAIN—AND TRUST

Every dentist has had cases that just didn't respond to anesthetic; the differentiator is how you deal with them. Sometimes, the problem is that the tooth is so infected and inflamed that it's just too sensitive to be worked on. When I come across a patient I can't numb in a situation like this, I will tell the patient, "Look, I'm going to try it one more time, but if this doesn't work, I'm afraid that this tooth will not get numb today. We need the tooth to settle down and we'll do this another day when I can numb you." I won't do the procedure, because dentistry should not be painful. When a dentist tells you, "You can't be feeling this," or, "I used a lot of anesthetic," or, least comforting of all, "Just hang on," the message they're really sending is, "You're a big baby—stop bothering me." To me, that's tantamount to verbal abuse and I wouldn't put up with it as a patient, much less use such a tactic on a patient.

Of all the patients I've had whose dental phobias were debilitating to them, the worst story is one that a woman patient shared with me; she had been a kidnap victim, and was raped and beaten for weeks until she was able to escape. She told my assistant about this to explain why she sometimes would get panic attacks with men, particularly if they were standing over her. I felt so badly for her, we did everything we could to help her to get the help she needed, and it took patience on everyone's part. I told her, "There will always be a woman in the room with us—you'll never be alone with me." We started slowly, with an appointment that was just for the exam, and no procedures. Next time, she got her teeth cleaned. By the third appointment, she was able to have a filling. She's had a very hard time, though, and even though she tells me, "Please never retire—I could never trust another dentist," there are visits when she just can't keep herself from shaking and we have to stop. Experiences like that are so debilitating for the patient that it's impossible for anyone who hasn't experienced it personally to really comprehend the damage it does. I'm just glad I can help her most of the time, and that she feels safe enough to keep coming in.

Very often with fearful patients, I'll tell them, "What I'd like us to accomplish today is just this one thing, the smallest filling on your plan. We're going to do that first. That way, you get to know me. I get to know how you'll react and we'll have a good visit. You'll get more confident." You always validate, understand, and express to them that you understand and you're not going to hurt them.

THE PROBLEM OF GAGGING

I mentioned the fear of gagging earlier, but I wanted to reiterate here, because the fear of gagging is a little different than these other kinds of fears and phobias. It's most often based on a physical response that becomes an emotional issue when the person becomes afraid of vomiting at the dentist's office. The gag reflex is a normal and natural thing and happens when something touches the back of your tongue or the roof of your mouth, causing a reflexive contraction. It's not a bad thing; in fact, it's the way that your body protects itself from swallowing foreign objects and helps to prevent you from choking.

In most people, the gag reflex isn't a problem, but for the 10–15 percent of folks who have a hypersensitive gag reflex,[3] it can become a problem. Even brushing the teeth can cause the person to gag. Sometimes, oatmeal or other soft foods can trigger it, and certainly having a dentist's tools or someone's hands in their mouth is daunting to someone with this issue. Being tilted back (as in the dental chair) is also very uncomfortable for someone with a hyperactive gag reflex.

---

3   Live Science Staff, "What is the Gag Reflex?" Live Science, August 1, 2012, https://www.livescience.com/34110-gag-reflex.html.

We've found a number of ways to help patients, though, and make it possible for them to get treatment.

First, we work on them with the chair in an upright position and have found that really helps. We also teach them breathing techniques that can help alleviate gagging. Surprisingly, we find that a pinch of salt under the tongue can help with this condition, and many of our patients use that method to damp down their gag reflex. And, of course, the intraoral scanner that has replaced sticky tooth impressions for the most part is a tremendous help for those who dreaded the tray of goop that used to be necessary for taking impressions.

But if your fear is that you'll vomit on the dentist, please rest assured that it won't be the first time—not by a long shot!—and if it's a problem for you, don't be afraid to let your dentist know and to ask for accommodations and suggestions.

TMJ ISSUES CAN CREATE FEAR, TOO

If something bad has happened to you in the past, then it's perfectly reasonable and normal to worry that it could happen again—and for some fearful patients whose TMJ issues have caused their jaws to dislocate when they opened wide, that becomes a reason to avoid seeing the dentist.

Because of the anatomy and the function of the temporomandibular joint, it's unique; it's not just your typical ball-and-socket joint that simply rotates, since people can also protrude their jaw. It's a rotating joint that also slides. And in that joint, between the two bones, is a thin cartilage, and the cartilage has to slide and rotate between the two joint pieces. Very often, the anatomy of the cartilage changes, and it begins to click or pop and causes pain. When the patient opens wide to eat a sandwich or to yawn, the jaw dislocates. Then, they can't close; someone has to push it back into place, and it hurts. They're afraid to open wide and to have treatment done because of their fear of a recurring dislocation.

For these patients, I can tell them, "I understand that. I've had that before. I know what you're talking about, and I'll make sure that we don't have you open that wide. We'll figure out a way to get your treatment done and not dislocate your jaw." Again, as long the dentist is aware of the issue, he or she should be able to work around it.

IS FEAR GENETIC? IN SOME CASES, THAT MAY BE TRUE!

It sounds like science fiction, but there is evidence that some dental fear may actually be genetically inherited. In studies done by researchers at the University of Pittsburgh and at West Virginia University, 1,370 subjects between the ages of eleven and seventy-four were surveyed in a family-based cohort study, measuring their dental fear and fear of pain.[4] In their findings, they say the data showed that, "dental fear was 30% heritable among those surveyed, and fear of pain was 34% heritable." The researchers also found "a substantial genetic correlation between dental fear and fear of pain, suggesting they are genetically related, though from distinct phenotypes."

> The researchers also found a substantial genetic correlation between dental fear and fear of pain, suggesting they are genetically related, though from distinct phenotypes.

Why would this be the case? The researchers suggest that the issue may be a tendency to feel pain more keenly than normal, or

---

4   C. L. Randall et al., "Toward a Genetic Understanding of Dental Fear: Evidence of Heritability," *Community Dent Oral Epidemiol* 45 (2017): 66–73.

that perhaps it involves having a higher-than-average flight-or-fight response that causes the person with that gene to react to stressful situations with panic more easily than does the average person. It's a fascinating field of study and may unlock many new therapies down the line for those whose genes are dictating their emotional responses.

That said, in my experience when we talk about "inherited" fear of the dentist, what we usually mean is that your family members talked about their fears or modeled them to you as a child, and you very naturally picked up the message that the dentist's office was a scary place, and dentists weren't to be trusted. Parents, if you're phobic, please do your very best not to share that with your children.

When I examine a child and I find a cavity, I take care to report it to the parent (and the child) in a very nonchalant, calming manner, saying: "This tooth has a cavity; next time I'll clean it." What the child hears is a calm voice, sounding like this "cavity" is very common and next time the dentist will "clean" it. It is presented such that the patient is not alarmed. I keep the tone light and easy. Unfortunately, at the moment I first mention that a cavity is present, the parent will gasp audibly, or say, "Oh no!" These reactions are certainly picked up by the child and the parent's fears are then "inherited." It is then that I take the parent aside and point out that their reactions are picked up by their child and will instill anxiety. I also let them know that performing the filling will truly be done in a way that will not hurt the child, so as to allow the child not fear going to the dentist in the future. I suggest that if they need to discuss the upcoming visit, they should use the same kind of relaxed tone of voice that I did, and just say that the tooth will be cleaned; and that if they

> Parents, please do not "prep" your child for dental appointments.

have more questions, they can ask the dentist.

Parents, please do not "prep" your child for dental appointments. You're going to say things that are going to be interpreted completely opposite of the way you intended them to be, and you are likely to undermine your child's sense of security. Instead, act nonchalant. Even if you yourself are an anxious patient, that's certainly not one of the things you want to pass on to your child.

Sometimes, an adult or an older sibling will tease a child about getting treatment— "Oh, that's gonna hurt!" or when they are going to receive and injection, they will tell the child that "It will only hurt for a second" —which creates the expectation of pain that leads to dental fears. Other times, we come across parents who have used threats of having to go to the dentist to bully their children into compliance about things like brushing their teeth or avoiding snacks. While we're all for good diet and good hygiene, scaring your child so much that they spend their adult lives avoiding dental care is not exactly the best way to insure their health.

Parents like to be with their children in the treatment room, and that's great—unless that parent uses the time to "joke" with the child about things that inspire fear. Usually, it's dads who are the worst culprits; they stand behind the child and say things like, "Whoa, look at the size of that horse needle!" or, "Here comes the drill!" Even a child who wasn't nervous going in is going to respond to that. That's when I invite the parent out into the hall and have "The Talk"; either he is going to quiet down and stop making the jokes, or he's going to have to wait in the waiting room. That's usually enough to hush him up, and we can get back to work.

CHILDREN ARE OFTEN AFRAID OF STRANGERS

Again, you can easily understand the basis for this kind of fear, because as parents we're constantly telling our kids to avoid contact—especially physical contact—with adults whom they don't know. Then we bring them into the dentist's office for the first time and wonder why they freak out when someone unfamiliar puts them in a chair and tells them to open their mouth!

The solution for the dentist is to win them over and gain their trust, to use one of the six principles of influence, in this case, getting them to like you.

When I walk in the room with a child, the first thing I do is look at them and say, "Oh, hi." Then, I turn to the parent and I totally ignore the child. I make sure I'm just talking to the parents for about two or three minutes. I want this kid to feel free to watch me and size me up a bit. If a child is shy and I try to jolly them out of it, chances are they'll just retreat further into shyness. But if I let them warm up at their own pace, they nearly always get over it. When I sense that they're feeling more comfortable, I'll turn to them and say something like, "Hey, I like your shoes. Those are cool shoes. Those are neat." I compliment them. When someone compliments you, you can't help being impressed with his good taste, and the child warms up to me. There are too many dentists out there who can't be bothered with this introductory step. They just want to numb the person, get the work done, and that's it: too bad if the patient is anxious. Unfortunately, that is a disservice to a patient. It makes their anxiety worse, and they will be less healthy in the long run because of it. When I work with a new child patient, I see it as an opportunity to help that child build a healthy, trusting relationship with me—and maybe keep them from developing dental anxiety as they get older. That's a big responsibility, and I take it seriously.

NO FEAR IS UNREASONABLE, ONCE YOU UNDERSTAND WHERE IT'S COMING FROM

In the previous chapter, Dr. Murphy described a patient who had what seemed like an unreasonable fear that her teeth were very weak and that any work on them would cause them to fall out. It sounds odd, until you know her backstory.

When she was younger, the patient had suffered an accident that had broken or cracked several of her teeth. They were repaired with a filling material. But the material used wasn't really suited to making such big repairs, and didn't last long, so over time, pieces of it came out, along with the broken teeth. No wonder she'd taken the notion that her teeth couldn't handle being worked on, or were too weak to hold a filling.

When showing her the x-rays of her teeth and reassuring her wasn't enough to make her feel better, I said, "I understand you're worried about that, and I promise you I'm going to be extra careful and gentle with those weak teeth." It was a way to reassure her and to validate her feelings—and that's more important to me than being "right."

No matter what the source of your dental fears or phobias may be, please don't let them stop you from seeking out the help you need. A caring dentist will understand, will take the time to validate your feelings, and will be willing and ready to help you to work through them. We're not here to judge you; we're here to get you healthy and keep you that way. Tell us what worries you have and what you're afraid of, and we're going to do everything we possibly

> No matter what the source of your dental fears or phobias may be, please don't let them stop you from seeking out the help you need.

can to make your experience as stress-free and comfortable as it can be.

Recently, I treated a patient whose teeth were severely worn down, to the extent that over 50 percent of her tooth structure was gone. If she didn't get treatment, she was on her way to losing all of her teeth. However, to save her teeth, the work would involve crowns on most of her teeth. This is the classic example of how a person's anxiety kept them from being able to go to the dentist and contributed to worsening of the health of their teeth to their point that they now need very extensive treatment. Also, knowing that their dental needs are so great causes their anxiety to heighten. Fortunately, we were able to counsel her, helped her focus on how we would be able to address her anxiety and be able to receive treatment. She now has teeth restored to their full size and she loves her new smile!

CHAPTER 3

The Benefits of Overcoming Dental Anxiety

Dr. Chris Murphy

If you suffer from dental anxiety, then you probably avoid the dentist for as long as you possibly can. You'll put up with pain and discomfort or live with a smile you have to hide behind closed lips or your hand—but you won't go to the dentist until an emergency like a painful abscess or a broken tooth drives you there. Common sense probably tells you that waiting until there's no other choice is not a healthy way to live—but somehow, you just can't bring yourself to make that call until agony forces your hand.

The biggest problem with going that route is that your mouth is not a discrete system that is disconnected to the rest of your body, but rather, an important part of the whole—and an infection there can rapidly turn into something very serious indeed—even life threatening. I was deeply saddened several years back to read the story of a twelve-year-old boy who died of a brain infection when his dental abscess was left untreated. In that case, his family's inability to access care was part of the problem—but those who choose not to get care can easily find themselves in the same situation. Infection doesn't stop with the infected tooth: it's just the jumping-off point. In another more recent case, an apparently healthy young man of twenty-six died when infection from his tooth spread to his heart and lungs—in only six days.

Yes, these are extreme examples—but hardly unique. Even in less dire circumstances, the damage to your health from poor oral care or poor oral hygiene can be great.

PERIODONTITIS IS MORE THAN BLEEDING GUMS

If you don't get regular cleanings, then you're a good candidate for periodontitis, even if you're careful about brushing and flossing. While the easiest-to-spot symptoms of gum disease, like swollen or sore gums that bleed easily, are painful, it's the problems you can't see that should worry you.

First is the danger to your teeth themselves. The sticky bacterial plaque that builds up on your teeth gets into your gums, creating that tell-tale reddening and inflammation, and can eventually cause some serious damage. If it's not removed by regular professional cleanings, the inflammation can spread along the roots of the teeth, causing destruction of the periodontal ligament and the supporting bone. That makes your teeth get loose, and eventually fall out—not good! And once you get past a certain point, there's just no saving them.

Once you lose the teeth, that's when the bone starts shrinking away, and eventually it can dissolve to the point where, when you open your mouth, your lower jaw fractures, because of the muscle attached to the lower jaw. At some point, if it's thin enough, the jaw will break on its own, or you'll get a slight bump in your face and your jaw will break.

I've actually had patients suggest that I should pull all of their teeth and replace them with dentures, so they'll never be bothered with them again. That's a bad idea, because when the teeth are gone, the bone begins to shrink—and you'll have nothing to hold your dentures with.

If you have significant gum disease, the bacteria in your mouth gets into your bloodstream. If you have an area like an artificial joint or artificial valve anywhere in your circulatory system that

> If you have significant gum disease, the bacteria in your mouth gets into your bloodstream.

disrupts the normal flow of blood, that bacteria flowing through your bloodstream can end up stuck in a spot where it's not a straight shot through the cardiac system, and infect that joint or valve. You end up with the risk of a heart condition that could prove to be fatal. The bacteria themselves cause hardening of the arteries (atherosclerosis), which causes heart attacks.[5] Your risk of a heart attack and cardiac issues is going to increase dramatically if you have bacteria chronically harboring in your mouth. And incidence of respiratory problems rises too—everything from pneumonia to COPD—in people with bad oral health.

Either chronic gum disease or a tooth abscess can spread these bacteria. Since a tooth abscess is going to cause pain, patients, even

---

5   James Beck et al., "Periodontal Disease and Cardiovascular Disease," *Jour. of Peridontology* 67, no. 105 (October 1, 1996): 1123–1137. https://doi.org/10.1902/jop.1996.67.10s.1123.

nervous ones, might come in and get the tooth extracted, in which case then the source of bacteria is gone. But if you already have gum disease, it's always there, you're always infected, and it's continuously doing damage.

Recent research has connected these same bacteria with a whole host of other life-threatening illnesses too, including stroke,[6] diabetes,[7] and even dementia.[8] And if you're pregnant, it's important to know that periodontitis has also been tied to low-birth-weight babies.

There's no reason any of this has to happen—because all it takes to prevent periodontitis is regular professional cleanings. But if you can't overcome your fear of the dentist to get there, then you're putting your health at risk.

ANOTHER CASUALTY OF BAD TEETH? YOUR NUTRITION

Do you find that chewing is painful? If you do, chances are that you are in the habit of only eating those things that don't challenge your teeth: soft foods and overcooked vegetables, for instance, over crispy raw vegetables, leafy greens, or fresh fruit. While it's possible to get adequate nutrition from soft foods, many people fall back on processed foods because putting that boiled chicken breast in the blender just isn't that appetizing. Processed foods tend to be high in sugar and in salt and eating them consistently puts your health at even greater risk.

By far, the most common and most damaging nutritional mistake that people make is to consume sugars as part of their daily

---

6   Armin J. Grau et al., "Periodontal Disease As a Risk Factor for Ischemic Stroke," *Stroke* 35 (2004): 496–501.

7   P. M. Preshaw et al., "Periodontitis and Diabetes: A Two-Way Relationship," Diabetologia 55, no. 1 (2012): 21–31. https://doi: 10.1007/s00125-011-2342-y. PMCID: PMC3228943.

8   Elizabeth Krall Kaye et al., "Tooth Loss and Periodontal Disease Predict Poor Cognitive Function in Older Men," *Am. Geriatrics Soc.* 58, no. 4 (2010): 713–718. https://doi.org/10.1111/j.1532-5415.2010.02788.x.

routine. In most cases, that consumption happens via beverages that people sip on throughout their day. People love to sip on beverages, especially if it's something sweet. However, this daily, repetitive appearance of sugar on your teeth gives the cavity-causing bacteria exactly the fuel they need to decay all of your teeth: sugar. This also happens if the patient uses breath mints with sugar each day, or gum with sugar. Please take stock of your daily routine and eliminate these sugars from your diet.

> Having to give up your favorite dishes because you can no longer chew them properly is no fun at all.

For most of us, food is one of life's real pleasures—and having to give up your favorite dishes because you can no longer chew them properly is no fun at all.

It's also important to note here that one of the major functions of chewing is to begin the digestive process. When you chew food, digestive enzymes in your saliva start to break down the food, helping your stomach to metabolize the foods you eat. When you can't chew, your body can't get the good out of what you do eat.

A DENTAL EXAM COVERS MORE THAN TEETH AND GUMS

Did you know that your dentist is the person who's most likely to spot oral cancers—and at their earliest stages?

Your general practitioner won't notice a growth in your mouth until it's pretty large, because, unlike dentists, doctors aren't familiar with what the normal mouth structure looks like. And by the time the cancer is large enough for them to detect it, it's more far advanced than you want it to be.

Mouth cancer is bad news. Not only is it typically a poor prognosis, but it's also very disfiguring if it gets too big. Nobody wants to end up missing part of their jaw after a "successful" surgery. I once spotted cancer in a very early stage under the tongue of one of my patients—but it took her weeks to follow up with her doctor as I'd advised her to do. Her surgery involved removing part of her skull. Had I not continued to push her to get to her doctor, she would have let it go. Early detection of disease is a big advantage of getting examinations of your mouth, especially for cancer. There are other things that can show up in your mouth that aren't pleasant, but oral cancer is the worst.

Chewing tobacco is very popular across a lot of the country, and there's been a rise on oral cancers concurrent with its rise in popularity. If you or someone you care about chews tobacco and isn't getting to the dentist twice a year for an exam, then you or they are effectively playing Russian roulette.

Cancer isn't the only kind of growth we discover in patients' mouths. I was doing free dentistry in the Solomon Islands once, and the doctor of one of the employees of the dive shop we were using as a makeshift treatment facility asked me to check him out. There was a tumor growing in his throat; the doctor had seen it but had written it off as a "normal" bony growth called *a tori*. People have them all the time, and it's usually associated with clenching and grinding. But it wasn't *a tori* and he had to have it removed.

PLEASE DON'T WAIT UNTIL YOU'RE IN PAIN

Too many people wait until they're in agony from an impacted tooth or an abscess before coming in to see a dentist. We can give them painkillers and antibiotics, but the fact is, if you've got one tooth that's killing you, it's likely that your other teeth also need attention and will eventually give you pain. Often, I find that someone who comes in with one tooth that's giving them extreme pain has others that are nearly as bad—and those start hurting as soon as the first one is taken care of. Why? The nerves can only handle so much stimulation, so it's difficult to differentiate the sources of the pain you experience when it's coming from multiple places. Sometimes, you'll feel what's called *referred pain*, which is pain that is felt in the body someplace other that its actual source. For instance, you might experience neck or back pain when the underlying cause is actually a bad tooth.

> Too many people wait until they're in agony from an impacted tooth or an abscess before coming in to see a dentist.

The same thing is true, of course, with people with multiple teeth that hurt. Once you take the most painful one out, you may not feel that much better, because now the other teeth are making themselves known. This happens all the time with folks whose teeth are in a bad way.

BAD TEETH HAVE OTHER COSTS, TOO— TO YOUR CAREER AND SOCIAL LIFE

We may not like it, and it isn't fair, but it's true nevertheless: people judge us by our appearance, and a bad appearance can cost you— literally. Your ability to climb the economic ladder and to compete with others for jobs is compromised if your teeth look bad, because honestly, nobody wants to interact with someone who looks like that. You're limiting your economic opportunities, particularly in any area in which your job requires you to interact with the public. Studies both here and abroad tell us what we know instinctively—that people make all kinds of assumptions about your education, your economic status, and your intelligence based on your teeth, and if they're bad or discolored or missing, then that judgment can be harsh.

In a study published by the *British Dental Journal*, researcher Peter Robinson showed one hundred and eighty female participants one of six images, either a male or a female digitally altered to display one of three possible dental statuses (unmodified, decayed, or whitened). The images were rated on four personality traits: social competence (SC), intellectual ability (IA), psychological adjustment (PA), and relationship satisfaction (RS).

The findings? "Decayed dental appearance led to more negative judgments over the four personality categories. Whitened teeth led to more positive appraisals. The gender of the image and the demographic background of the participant did not have a significant effect on appraisals." Robinson concludes, "Tooth color exerts an influence on social perceptions. The results may be explained by negative beliefs about dental decay, such as its link with poor oral hygiene." White teeth made people seem to be smarter, better adjusted, and more attractive—while discolored teeth evoke the opposite.[9]

One of my patients was a very competent driver with a local shuttle bus company who was told by his supervisor that people were reacting negatively to his appearance; he had missing and discolored teeth, and apparently, there had been complaints; riders saw him as less than competent and perhaps even untrustworthy, because of his appearance. He had to fix his teeth in order to keep his job. I was able to do a nice-looking restoration on his teeth, and he was able to continue in his position.

And studies also show that we like and trust people who smile

---

9   Peter G. Robinson, "The Influence of Tooth Colour on the Perceptions of Personal Characteristics Among Female Dental Patients: Comparisons of Unmodified, Decayed and 'Whitened' Teeth," *British Dental Journal* 204 (March 2008): 256–257.

at us—and don't warm up to those who do not. As evidenced by a study done at the University of Wyoming, it was a woman's smile that was the biggest predictor of whether someone looking at her found her likeable and attractive—not her body posture. And the wider the smile, the more attractive she appeared.[10]

Bad breath (halitosis) is another problem associated with poor oral health and hygiene—and that's certainly a popularity killer, no matter how old you are.

YOUR SELF-ESTEEM TAKES A HIT, TOO

Even if you're willing to dismiss what anyone else thinks of you, there's still the erosion of your self-esteem that happens every time you catch sight of your teeth in a mirror. Most of us get good at not really "seeing" ourselves, with our mind's eye editing out the parts of ourselves we don't like very much. But when we *do* look, really look, and see ourselves as others do, it wears us down if the person looking back at us in the mirror has ugly teeth. What's amazing to me, though, and part of the reason I love my work, is that when that bad smile is repaired, the patient's self-esteem goes through the roof. It's great to see.

One woman in particular stays in my memory: She was a very fearful patient and had serious issues with her back teeth, several of which required crowns. Her front teeth were discolored and unattractive, but I was more concerned initially with getting her teeth fully functional than I was with improving her looks. Still, I suggested that we might try some veneers to enhance her appearance after the back teeth were finished, and offered to put temporaries on for her so she could wear them home and try them out. She agreed, and I put them on.

---

10   Hugh McGinley, Patsy McGinley, and Karen Nicholas, "Smiling, Body Position, and Interpersonal Attraction," *Bulletin of the Psychonomic Society* 12. (1978): 21-24. 10.3758/BF03329613.

About an hour after she left the office, my assistant came to tell me that the woman was on the phone, and she was crying. *What in the world—had the temporaries fallen off?*

I took the call, and the woman was still sobbing. She managed to tell me, though, that she'd never, ever thought in her life that she could look so good—and that when she'd gotten home and smiled at herself in the mirror for the first time in years, the change in her appearance just overwhelmed her. She couldn't stop thanking me—and these were just the temporaries! "I felt ugly for so long!" she said. Honestly, I still choke up when I think about that, and what a difference it made in her whole personality. When she came for the permanent veneers, she was bubbly and thrilled to show off that new smile. She just blossomed. It really changed her life, and it was beautiful to see.

Another patient whose transformation was like night and day was Ella, a shy, diffident woman who first came to see me when she was in her twenties. She was embarrassed by her teeth—or rather, by her lack of them; she was wearing a removable denture with the four front teeth in it. Her body language as I talked with her was completely closed and withholding, and I could see by the way she dropped her head when she spoke that this was a long-standing problem, because her whole personality was so withdrawn. I asked her how she had lost so many teeth when she was so young.

She told me, "I fell when I was seven. I was up on a counter, and I was getting cookies out of the cupboard. I backed up a little bit and slipped right off the counter with my mouth open, and hit the counter on the way down on my front teeth and broke them off."

That was shocking—but not as shocking as what she told me next. I asked her, "When did you get that partial plate?"

It turns out that she didn't get it until she was over age eighteen—and she told me that she had gone all through her childhood and high school years without her front teeth. Can you imagine how tough that must have been on a sensitive young girl? I myself had knocked my front tooth hard enough when I was about twelve years old to turn it brown, and the embarrassment of that is something I still can't recall without cringing. For Ella, it must have been so much worse.

Ella had other more pressing issues that had finally brought her into the office, but I said, "Do you really like that partial? Because you could have something you didn't have to take out, or I could make you a bridge," and she wasn't sure. She liked the idea, but had no idea what a difference it would make in her life. Long story short, I made her the bridge, cemented it in, and it looked great.

She came back to the office six months later, and she was a different person. She was smiling; she looked at me when she spoke, and her body language was noticeably far more relaxed. Clearly, the damage done to her psyche by what she'd gone through was deep, but I could see she was so much better already. Honestly, if I'd been her dad, I'd have moved heaven and earth to help her when the accident had happened all those years back. I was glad I could help her now.

PLEASE DON'T LET YOUR LIFE AND HEALTH BE DIMINISHED BY YOUR FEARS

> No matter how fearful you are, please believe me—to go on risking your health and happiness because of your fears and phobias is dangerous and self-destructive.

Whether we're talking about your physical health or your mental health, every study I've read and every interaction I've had with patients tells me that having bad teeth has a damaging impact on people; that ugly, discolored teeth can hold you back in life in every way, and make you terribly self-conscious and self-hating.

No matter how fearful you are, please believe me—to go on risking your health and happiness because of your fears and phobias is dangerous and self-destructive. There is help, and there are caring professionals who understand how you feel, who will do everything they can to get you past your fears and on the right track.

CHAPTER 4

Self-Esteem and How Others See You

Dr. Scott Billings

When we let ourselves go, it's usually a gradual progress, not a dramatic change—so it's easy for us to lose sight of how we've come to look, or how we appear to others. But when it's something as noticeable as our teeth, it's tough for us to ignore, and that takes a toll on our self-esteem and confidence.

Smiling is a reflexive, natural way to express friendliness, interest, amusement, or affection—and when we have to cover our smile, or lose the habit of smiling altogether, it makes it harder to connect with others, because they're likely to see us as cold and standoffish. As you've seen, a smile that is not appealing damages our career prospects, because we look less intelligent or less educated than we are. Bad teeth, missing teeth, or discolored teeth can also make us look older than our age, and can cause our cheeks to sag, creating lines and hollows in our faces.

In the previous chapter, Dr. Murphy talked about the research studies that reveal how quickly (and often cruelly) we're judged on our appearance—but the self-judgment is just as bad if not worse, because every time we catch sight of our ugly smile, it chips another little piece off of our self-esteem. We feel less lovable, less strong, less desirable, less appealing—just *less* than we actually are. And that gets worse as we get older.

Sometimes, it will take someone else speaking honestly to a person to make them realize how they look, or that they don't smile. A patient of mine came in with a complaint about his appearance; one of his front teeth was set far back, and whenever he got his picture taken, he'd noticed that it made him look as though he was missing a tooth. Someone had pointed out to him that he never smiled—and he'd realized that was true. It was a habit he'd developed to hide that tooth. He didn't want to go through life as the guy who never smiles? So we did some cosmetic work to make the teeth straight. He was delighted with the results—and his smile came back. It was as though his whole demeanor brightened up.

Another of my patients is a schoolteacher, who started out as a very anxious patient. He avoided dentists and only came to see me because he was about to lose his front tooth. Unfortunately, the tooth could not be saved—but I was able to alleviate his anxiety by letting him know that we could have a replacement tooth made and placed immediately, so that he wouldn't have to go home with a gap where his front tooth should have been. Subsequently, he was able to get some restorative work done. As a teacher, he just couldn't stand the thought of being in front of his classes with a missing front tooth. Once he felt better about the way we treated him, he started coming in regularly, and the improvement to his appearance really made him feel great about himself. He's a far happier and more confident guy than he was when I first met him.

WE SUPPORT OUR PATIENTS THROUGHOUT THEIR PROCESS

A woman executive came to me for help; her twenty-year-old bridge was an embarrassment to her because it was dark and chipped and she felt that it made her look less professional. She had a mouthful of crowns, too, that weren't the right colors, and when she smiled, it frankly ruined all the care she'd put into making her appearance that of a person in an important executive position. She was otherwise lovely, very well dressed and coiffed, but that unsightly smile just didn't fit in with the rest of her. She'd gotten into the habit of covering her mouth or turning away when she smiled, but she knew that people noticed, and she was understandably worried that it was keeping her from moving up in her job. She was expected to interact with the public and to do presentations for her peers and her bosses, and she couldn't continue to dodge those meetings without damaging her prospects. Like so many of our patients, she had dental anxiety and had put off the work she needed for a long time. But she'd finally had enough, and was ready to brave the chair.

I praised her courage, because I know how tough it is for someone to put their fears aside and come in. I talked to her about how much better she'd feel once it was done, and walked her through feeling embarrassment because of the condition of her teeth. Our anxious patients have an even bigger issue, because on top of that, they're worried that a dentist will think less of them for being fearful. But when you take care of your teeth, that self-esteem problem, along with that feeling of being embarrassed about either your teeth or your anxiety, is going to go away. Whether your teeth are broken or missing, brown, or out of alignment—once you steel yourself to take that first step of coming into the office, we can help you, not only with your teeth but also with your anxiety.

When you work in a business or industry in which appearance is a major factor, it's important to do everything you can to make sure you're competitive. One of my patients was a newscaster on a national network; her teeth weren't as big or bright as they should have been, and she had very real concerns about the effect that might have on her television career, given how much emphasis is put on appearance in that line of work. I did veneers on all six of her front teeth, making them lighter and a better shape, and creating much more pleasing proportions. She was thrilled about it, and I could see how much she enjoyed sharing that new smile.

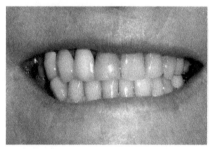 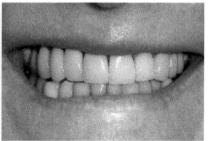

BEFORE   AFTER

NEW TECHNOLOGY MAKES IT SO EASY TO HAVE A GREAT SMILE

There are so many great options available now for people whose teeth present a bad appearance. Spacing or coloring problems can be solved with veneers and bleaching, bringing optimal spacing and brightness to your smile. These are quick and easy procedures that make a tremendous difference. Sometimes I see a patient who needs a denture because their front teeth have given out after years of neglect. I can't tell you how amazing the transformation is when someone gets a whole new set of front teeth, and the response when they get that first look in the mirror. They literally sob with joy, because now they have a beautiful smile again. That's what makes my work so satisfying—and I enjoy seeing them so happy that I tend to tear up a bit myself.

> I can't tell you how amazing the transformation is when someone gets a whole new set of front teeth.

I had a fifteen-year-old patient who came in to see me because she was going to be getting braces. She had what's called "peg laterals," a common deformity of the front lateral incisors, which are the teeth on each side of the front middle two top teeth. When they're disproportionately small, they're called peg laterals, and hers were really tiny. We had the orthodontist position all her other teeth correctly; then, when her orthodontic treatment was finished, we put veneers on those little peg laterals so they looked full and proportionate to the rest of her teeth. Now, after going through her childhood with tiny, crooked teeth, she has a beautiful, full smile. How much difference do you think that will make in her life as she goes forward? I'd say a lot; research also shows that pre-teens and teens that have ugly teeth carry the burden of low self-esteem with them throughout their lives.

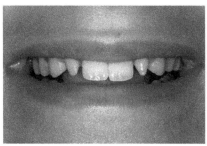 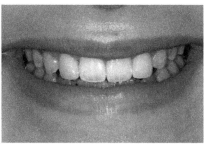

BEFORE   AFTER

Sometimes, it's a special occasion that prompts a patient to finally get their smile fixed—a wedding, for instance, or a family reunion where they'll be encountering people they have not seen for years. I treated a woman who was going to her fiftieth high school reunion, where she'd see old friends with whom she'd long been out of touch. She had always hated the spaces between her teeth and how dark they were, and that her bottom teeth were crooked. She was sixty-eight years old, and her husband had questioned why she'd choose to fix her teeth now, but as she told me, "It's time. I've waited all my life, always putting everyone and everything ahead of myself. I've been putting this off for years, so now, I'm doing it." We fixed her issues with a set of lovely crowns, and she went to that reunion with her smile restored. When she came back, she told me, "It was the best night I ever had."

One thirteen-year-old came to us because only four of her lower teeth were permanent teeth. She had five other teeth still there, but they were baby teeth and very small in proportion to the permanent teeth. She'd never lost those baby teeth, since the permanent teeth weren't under them to push them out. She was not a candidate for implants, though, because her bone was too thin. I told her parents, "We can make her a bridge." There was risk involved, as I explained to them ahead of time; if the baby teeth were to develop problems down the line, then we wouldn't be able to do root canals or take other measures to save them. That meant that we might end up having to do further work in years to come, or replace the bridge. But they could see how unhappy their little girl was with her appearance, so they decided to go ahead. I made her a ten-tooth fixed bridge that went all the way around from left to right, what we call a *roundhouse bridge*. Now she has teeth that stay in, and they're beautiful. It's been a year and a half and she hasn't had any problems. It means so much to her, to feel normal and happy about her appearance. I don't think there's a more important investment in her future happiness that her parents could have made.

WHEN YOUR LIFE HITS A CROSSROAD

Sometimes, people find themselves at turning points in their lives that makes them finally take action to improve their smiles. The loss of a job, the loss of a spouse, or the end of a long-term relationship—any of these major life changes can provide the impetus that folks need to make them finally commit to doing something good for their appearance. A divorce can be devastating to someone's self-esteem, and the thought of entering the dating pool after a certain age is frankly terrifying for many people. Some time ago, a divorced woman came in to see me; she told me that she'd just cashed her settlement check, and she was there to get her teeth done; she said, "I'm treating myself!"

She confided that it had been a tough breakup and hard on her confidence. Now, she wanted to give herself a boost of confidence, because she wanted to start dating—and couldn't stand the way her teeth looked when she smiled. She was very happy with the results. In fact, just fixing her smile created a kind of cascade effect for her. Now, she wanted to

> Often people who've more or less given up on how they look have that attitude turned around when their smiles are rejuvenated.

lose weight, to work out, and to change how she did her hair. Over the months that followed, we saw her looking younger, better, and happier—and it all started with a great smile. That's not uncommon; often people who've more or less given up on how they look have that attitude turned around when their smiles are rejuvenated.

Want more proof that a great smile can help your love life—and that a bad one undermines you? Match.com did a survey of about 5,500 single adults on what mattered most to them in a potential mate—and good teeth topped the list of important qualities.[11] About two-thirds of the men in the survey reported that they felt that good teeth were the most important factor in judging the attractiveness of a potential date. And nearly three-quarters (71 percent) of the women interviewed said they ranked the state of a man's teeth as the first consideration in deciding whether or not to date them! A biological anthropologist who helped the company develop the survey, Dr. Helen Fisher, observed that the results weren't surprising, because the state of our teeth is a reflection of the state of our health—an important factor in choosing a mate.

> No patient of mine has to settle for "good enough," and you shouldn't either.

Nearly all of our patients are delighted with the work they get; to be honest, it's usually the dentist who will say, "I want to tweak that just a bit" because we see flaws where the patient just sees a great result. It's funny to have to argue with someone who's telling you, "No, no. I look fine." But fine isn't the same thing as great, and I'm going for more than fine. I usually succeed in overruling them, and when we're done, it *does* look great. No patient of mine has to settle for "good enough," and you shouldn't either.

---

11   Sharon Jayson, "What Singles Want: Survey Looks at Attraction, Turn-Offs," *USA Today*, February 5, 2013, www.usatoday.com/story/news/nation/2013/02/04/singles-dating-attraction-facebook/1878265/.

DON'T GIVE UP ON YOURSELF!

Don't dismiss yourself as being beyond help. There's a lot we can do with very little tooth. We have patients who come in and say, "You've got to pull this tooth, I know you won't be able to save it." It's probable that they've put off coming in, because nobody really wants a tooth pulled. They're always astonished when we're able to tell them, "No, we *can* save that tooth." I've seen patients come in with damaged teeth that were flat to the gum line—but we could actually build the tooth up and restore the tooth, finishing the procedure with a crown. Once the MIA tooth is back in business, they don't have an ugly gap to contend with.

Sometimes, even people who work with dentists put off getting cosmetic treatment, even though they know how much it would help them. My favorite example of that is my dental hygienist's husband—who owns a dental lab. He makes crowns, and very good ones; he'd had unsightly gaps between his teeth his whole life, and finally decided to do something about it. I took his tooth impressions, and he made his own crowns. I installed them for him, and now he looks great—no more gaps. Better yet, he uses those great-looking crowns as a sales tool; when he goes into make a call on a dentist who's looking to work with a new lab, he flashes his new smile and tells them, "I made these!"

A SMILE'S A TERRIBLE THING TO LOSE

So many things can happen over time to ruin the look of a smile. Often, people come in with fillings that have turned brown over the years, or with teeth that are worn down due to grinding or a bad bite. Teeth can get crooked over time, too, even if you started out with straight teeth. And, of course, many people, particularly those who avoid going to the dentist, do lose teeth as they get older.

Aging is challenging enough to our vanity without the added

psychological burden of having ugly teeth and having to hide your smile. If you catch yourself wincing when you look at your teeth, whether in the mirror or in a photo, or if you're suffering self-consciousness because you know others are reacting to how you look—or, worst of all, if you're in the habit of "smothering" your smile, or just have given up smiling all together—please know that there is compassionate help available. We can give you the smile you've always wanted or restore the one you lost over time.

But the first step is coming in—and that's one we hope you'll take. We'll meet you more than halfway.

CHAPTER 5

How We Give Power
Back to the Patient

Dr. Chris Murphy

I f you're a fearful or anxious patient, one of the hardest things about going to the dentist has to be the sense that you're rendered powerless once you're in that dental chair—that everything that happens from there on is in the dentist's hands, and nobody is going to pay attention to your wishes or to what you're feeling. That's a terrifying feeling, and one we certainly understand. That's why we do everything we can to give power back to our patients, and to ensure that they're the ones who call the shots when they're in our offices. It's all part of our philosophy of empowering them, which is the first step to helping those whose fears have kept them from getting the care they need.

In fact, every aspect of the care you get from us and from our assistants is informed by that view, from the way the receptionist welcomes you, to our techniques, and how our assistants are trained. That's why we have such an enviable record of success in working with fearful patients, and in turning them into fearless patients.

In our very first conversation, I always tell my new patients, "You don't need to be ashamed about being anxious. You don't have to be embarrassed about how your teeth look. I know that your anxiety is something you can't help, and you don't need to feel ashamed of it. I'm here to help you get the treatment you need, and we'll do it at your pace." I find that really helps to reassure people, because they realize that they finally have a dentist that understands them.

I always ask at what point they tend to become anxious; does worrying about the dentist keep them up the night before, or is getting a shot what they're afraid of, for instance. Their answers let me know what to expect and how and when I can best help them.

> If you're a fearful patient, it's as though you have a ball and chain around your ankle that contains all the weight of your negative past experiences with dentists and getting treatment.

We understand that it's tough to make that choice; if you're a fearful patient, it's as though you have a ball and chain around your ankle that contains all the weight of your negative past experiences with dentists and getting treatment. When I let them know that I'm different, and that my approach is all about making them feel safe, that shackle falls off and they can get into the dental chair.

WE'RE CAREFUL WITH CHILDREN

We understand that very often, the anxious patient developed that anxiety because of a bad experience they had in childhood. We certainly don't want to create any of those traumatizing memories for our young patients, and we recognize how important it is to have great technique when treating kids. We've standardized those techniques and trained everyone within our practice in them, to be sure everyone on the team understands and follows our protocols.

For instance, many children are afraid of the needle used to deliver anesthetic. If I have a child in the chair with the hygienist, and I find out they have a cavity, I'll say, "You've got some cavity germs on your tooth and we're going to clean that tooth next time, and fill it for you." I keep my tone very nonchalant and off-handed, so they know that it's no big deal. And I always take the parent aside to warn them against doing anything or saying anything that will color that child's expectations about the treatment he or she is going to get. I don't need parents "prepping" their kids with words and phrases they don't fully understand and that are going to strike fear into that child's heart.

If the child asks Mom or Dad what's going to happen, all the parent is going to say is, "Dr. Billings is going to clean and fill your tooth." If they ask more questions, the parents can tell the child to ask me. Why do I prep the parents? Because if I don't, they're likely to say stuff like, "Well, it only hurts for a minute." That's not going to reassure the child; they're going to be worrying that "He's going to hurt me!" It's horrible for them and for us, because they're scared before they even get here.

When I have to use anesthetic with children, I tell them we're going to put some sleepy juice on their tooth. That's a nice, simple phrase that tells them everything they need to know, because they understand that their tooth is going to go to sleep so that we can clean it and the child won't feel it.

Before I give them the shot, I tell them, "When I do this, you might feel a little pinch for a second. But it's only for a second, so it's easy." I'm pretty good at giving injections, and very often they won't feel it at all—but I like to prepare them by telling them the truth, because that helps them to trust me and to relax. "I'm telling you so you won't be surprised if it does pinch," goes a long way to building that trust.

Then I tell them, "And if you do feel a little pinch, all you have to do is raise your hand like this" —and I show them how, which is to flip their left hand up— "and that means stop, and I'll stop."

Once they're clear on that, I continue, "Okay, I'm going to put the sleepy juice on, and you might feel that little pinch." And then I go ahead and do it, adding, "I want you to raise your hand." So usually I place one drop of anesthetic and then I stop. When they raise their hand, I've already stopped, and they don't feel it anymore after that, because the needles we use nowadays are so small and so sharp. What hurts when they're getting the injection is actually not the needle, but the sting caused by the anesthetic solution. The local anesthetics are slightly acidic, so when you put that under the skin, it stings. After I put that first drop in, it starts to numb up the site—then I tell them, "Okay, I'm going to put another drop in, so you might feel a little pinch." And I actually put in a drop and I stop. Sometimes they raise their hand, and sometimes they don't, then I let that soak in. It only takes about five seconds to take effect, so by the third time, nearly all of them have stopped raising their hand. I always stop when they do, though, because I want them to understand they're in charge, and I respect their feelings. I make sure that they know I see their hand, and I don't ignore it. They get done, and they don't even know that they had a needle in there.

They just know they had sleepy juice. And they're fine.

As a matter of fact, I use the exact same technique with my adult patients (although I don't call it sleepy juice). If they feel the pinch, they raise their hand, and I stop. That small act of handing back control helps many people who are afraid of needles get past their nervousness.

Sometimes when I'm working with a child, it's the parent who is really the fearful one, and having that parent in the treatment room with their child can complicate things. One woman who was in the room with her son kept echoing my instructions; I'd say, "Okay, Sam, open up—" and she'd jump in with, "Open up, Sam!" We went along like that for a while, until I gently but firmly requested, "Sam can't listen to both of us at once, and he needs to focus on me right now. If you could, please just hold his hand—you don't have to speak, he knows you're here."

Sometimes, all it takes to get a really fearful child through a procedure is one of our great assistants coaching them through it and encouraging them. They're terrific at that.

> Sometimes, all it takes to get a really fearful child through a procedure is one of our great assistants coaching them through it and encouraging them. They're terrific at that.

When I see a child is really frightened, sometimes it's clear that trying to complete the procedure that particular day may well traumatize the patient. However, instead of just stopping I'll say, "I'm going to do one more thing and then we're done if you can do this."

They'll always say, "All right, one more thing." Then, when they open their mouth, I use the slow speed drill and just lightly rub it on a tooth's enamel; it doesn't do anything except vibrate, so they feel something touching their tooth.

At that point I'll say, "That was great, you did such a good job. All done for today." My assistant and I give the child praise and then send them home. We'll schedule them to come back the next week, saying: "Okay, we're going to do that again, it was so easy, right?" That really helps build their confidence, and suddenly they're not fearful anymore. Again, it takes patience and a real willingness to stop when the patient needs you to—and the sensitivity to know when that point has been reached.

WE UNDERSTAND FEAR OF NEEDLES

When I have a patient who's really phobic about needles, I tell them, "I understand there's a fear of needles and that needles can pinch, but I have a great technique. I'm going to share it with you, and I promise that this will be the best needle you've ever had in your life." Then, I explain about the acidity and how it's that first pinch that hurts—and if I let that soak in, by the time I put in the third drop, they're not going to feel anything because they'll be numbed. Every patient tells me, "That was the easiest shot I ever had." That starts the process of alleviating their anxiety.

Some patients, particularly children, come in so spooked about needles that giving them anesthetic can be quite challenging. Even though I've told them everything I'm going to do, in spite of all my preparation, they know it's coming and they panic; they raise their hand, or they turn their head. I refer to that as the "Moment of Truth."

When we come to that moment, either with a child or an adult patient, I go over that Moment of Truth with them. I say, "I know you're anxious, I know this is hard. It's your anxiety stopping you.

The anxiety is actually worse than the injection. So, let's do this; let's practice the Moment of Truth. I'm going to take this needle and bring it up to your mouth, but I'm not going to touch you with it. I'm just going to hold it there and then I'm going to take it away. When you're okay with that, we're going to put it right next to your gum, but I'm not going to touch your gum. And we're going to practice that. And then, when we actually go to do it, it's going to be easy."

After the third or fourth successful practice round, I'll say, "Now this time I'm going to inject for a second and stop. And you might feel a little pinch and that's going to be it, but I'm telling you it's going to be that easy." Very often, this is all it takes to get them past that Moment of Truth anxiety, and they discover that getting the injection isn't nearly as bad as they'd remembered or as they thought it was going to be.

Sometimes with older kids who are afraid of the needle, I'll ask them if they want to see it. They'll say, "Yeah." And I'll hold it in my hand where they can see it, and I'll flick the end of the needle itself, and say, "It's really flexible, it's soft, and it's not bad." And I'll squirt some of the anesthetic out: "It's like a squirt gun. You want to try?" And I actually let them hold the needle and squirt it. They get a kick out of that; they think that's hilarious. Very often, that's enough to give them the confidence to get past their fear and to let me go ahead.

WE ALWAYS STOP WHEN YOU ASK US TO STOP

Another technique I've found that helps people to get past their initial fear is to ask them about their previous experiences with dentists, particularly the ones that made them fearful. When they've told their story, I can reassure them that this time is going to be different, and explain how. Often, their issues sprung from a dentist who had

55

promised to stop if they were feeling pain, but in fact pressured them into continuing when they signaled him to stop. I can tell them, "I'd never do that. You are the boss. When you raise your hand, I'll stop every time. If you tell me that you're feeling it, I am going to numb it some more. Then, if you still feel it, I'm going to stop." I explain I've had occasions where we have tried to numb a tooth, but some reason,

> I'm so serious about not inflicting pain on them that I'll happily send them home and reschedule rather than doing so.

the tooth was very active and resisted getting numb. When that happens, I stop the procedure, put a temporary filling in or whatever I need to do, and tell the patient, "We're going to try this another day when the inflammation has gone down. We're going to do this the easy way." I can see a nervous patient relax when I explain that to them, because now they understand that I'm so serious about not inflicting pain on them that I'll happily send them home and reschedule rather than doing so.

Every fearful patient presents unique challenges; some of my patients find the whole notion of being in a dentist's office so terrifying that they can't even come in for the initial appointment. My assistant calls them and basically talks them down off the ledge, and we keep that supportive, positive talk up when they do come in. Once, when I was in dental school, a child I was getting ready to work on jumped up out of the chair and took off running. I had to chase him down the halls and into the waiting room, where about two hundred people were treated to the spectacle of a dental student chasing a screaming kid. They must have wondered what in the world I'd done to him, but we hadn't even started yet. My adult patients don't run from the room, but many of them do ask me to stop for a minute—or fifteen—when we're doing their work, and, of course, I always do.

We have one patient who brings a whole bag of comfort objects with her whenever she comes in: a blanket, a stuffed toy, and all kinds of other things. They work for her, and you know what? Giving power back to the patient means doing whatever it takes to make her comfortable, and that is perfectly fine with us. Whether you want a security blanket, your spouse, or one of our assistants to hold your hand—you can have it, and you don't need to feel shy about it.

In designing our offices and treatment rooms, we've made choices specific to comforting the fearful patient. Our ceilings are extra-tall, so claustrophobic patients feel more comfortable. Our treatment room chairs are made of memory foam and have such a fantastic heat and massage option built into them that our patients often ask us where they can get one to take home. There are televisions mounted on the ceiling, and noise-cancelling headphones. We have lovely throw blankets handy, and if someone looks chilly, we don't ask them if they want one, because people are so polite they don't want to trouble you, we just hand them one and say, "I thought you looked like you might be cold." We have water bottles on hand for patients, and lip balm in every room. We either offer that to them, or just say during treatment, "You know, your lips look dry, so I'm going to put this lip balm on for you." We even have special sunglasses so that when the patient is in the chair and leaning back, the light isn't going to bother their eyes. Everything is geared to providing comforts people want but might be too shy to ask for.

Every treatment room has a Wi-Fi speaker in it that communicates with the room's work station. The speaker program features all types of music; everything from Adele to Bach, with curated playlists by Pandora and SiriusXM. People really relax when they can listen to their favorite music.

We also take frequent breaks with anxious patients, so they have a chance to collect themselves and relax. Every ten or twenty seconds I'll stop, let them spit and catch their breath, and then we do a little more.

OUR ASSISTANTS HAVE GREAT PEOPLE SKILLS

We hire and train for great people skills for every person in our practice, because we find that anxious patients often feel safer and less embarrassed when talking to one of the team about what they need or how they're feeling. We give our assistants time to be in with the patient and bolster their confidence with the patient, so the patient feels the assistant is their advocate. Whether that means holding their hand when they're having an injection, or serving as their cheerleader during treatment—"You're doing so well!" or saying to me, "Let's stop for a minute, we're taking special care of her"—it provides a tremendous boost to a patient to have a staff member who's so clearly on their side. We do our training on this in-house; much of enlisting their help is just letting them know that it's welcome and valued, as sometimes an assistant will feel uneasy interceding for a patient because they don't want to get in the doctor's way. We make sure they understand that's exactly what we want them to do—that, in fact, patient comfort is their first priority.

> Our patients love our assistants so much that they'll request appointments when that assistant is available.

We train them on terminology, so that they don't use terms like "injection" or "shot" around the patient, and we train them on our techniques. We have a special way that, when they pass the anesthetic syringe, it's done in a smooth, quick hand-off. That way, we can go from taking the topical anesthetic out of the patient's mouth and putting the injection in without them seeing the needle first. We do let them know it's coming—no unpleasant surprises—but we don't want to wave it in front of them.

Our patients love our assistants so much that they'll request appointments when that assistant is available. I have a patient that we've been treating who required crowns on every tooth; she loves our assistant Jo, and she only wants Jo there when she comes, because she knows Jo is on her side and she trusts her. Sometimes, making sure that a particular assistant is there for the patient who needs her is a little challenging for us, because of staffing—but we never say no.

WORKING WITH THE PATIENT WHO GAGS EASILY

There are a few ways we can help our gagging patients; one is by teaching them simple breathing techniques that really help. When we are doing a procedure with the drill, water squirts out of it to keep the tooth cool. That water can fill up the back of the throat and stir up the gag reflex. But the patient breathes in and out in short, quick puffs through their nose, it stops the gagging response and they don't feel like they're choking. We call it *bunny breathing*, and it really works.

For a gagger, another great way to help them get through it is to have them sit up straight, then raise up one leg then put that down, then raise the other. That distraction is enough to make the gag reflex stop.

SPECIAL ISSUES

We see a wide variety of patients, some of whom have really unusual and specific issues. One of our patients has an allergy to certain kinds of plastics. These plastics cause her to get painful ulcerations in her mouth, so naturally she's anxious about being exposed to them. That meant we had to do a pretty deep dive, researching which plastics had that effect, and we've actually avoided using certain things that we normally use.

We have other patients who are very fearful about accidentally swallowing things during a procedure, bits of a filling, for instance. We've used rubber dams to avoid that, or sometimes make a sort of miniature net out of a piece of gauze and tucked it in over the tongue and around where we're working, so that nothing can get past it into the throat—a literal safety net!

We have patients who fear that their mouth will hurt or cramp when they have to hold it open too long. We have mouth props—little foam wedges—that allow these patients to rest their jaw. It keeps their mouth open without putting strain on the muscles.

I have patients who, because of either gagging issues or fear of swallowing, want to have their treatment done while they're sitting up straight. It's a little more difficult for me to work in that position, because it's harder to see into their mouth without bending myself like a pretzel—but I'm able to do it, as long as I don't have too many patients in a row that require it.

Some patients really don't care for those little suction tips we call *saliva ejectors*. Hygienists like to hang those over the corner of the patient's mouth when they're doing a cleaning, but these patients prefer to spit. We don't have cuspidors any more—they're a thing of the past—so we just hand the saliva ejector over to the patient and tell them they can hold it, put it in when they need to, and take it out when they don't want it.

WE'RE A PATIENT-CENTRIC PRACTICE

Whenever we're contemplating a change at the office—whether that's bringing in new technology, doing a new kind of training, or offering a new service—the question we ask first is, "What does that do for our patient? How does that make the patient's experience better?" Every choice we make is about creating a better and more supportive environment for our patients, one in which even the most phobic patient can relax, knowing they won't be hurt or shamed—and knowing that control over their experience is firmly in their hands.

CHAPTER 6

Medication Options for the Fearful Patient

Dr. Scott Billings

For those patients who just can't face dental treatment without medication, we offer a wide range of solutions, suited to almost every level of anxiety.

NITROUS OXIDE

Among the most popular of these is the gas nitrous oxide, because it's easily administered, takes effect very quickly, and wears off very rapidly, too—within three or four minutes—so the patient is able to drive themselves home or go back to work.

It produces what's called *mild sedation*, because you're awake and always aware of where you are and you're able to respond to requests, but you're in a pleasantly dreamy state that allows you to ignore what's going on around you. It's perfect for anxious patients, because for so many it stops that wave of anxiety that occurs as the dentist begins the procedure.

Most people can tolerate nitrous, though a very few (about 5 percent) may feel nauseous. And it's not something you have to plan for in advance. If you're in the chair and decide you need it, we can administer it on the spot; no fasting or any other preparation is required. That makes it a good solution for patients who didn't think they were going to be anxious but are beset with anxiety once they're in the chair.

The patient receives the nitrous oxide through a nasal mask, and we monitor their response, because, although you can't "overdose" on it, too much can produce delusions or an emotional response, so we'll continuously check in with the patient to make sure they're feeling as they should. Some people don't like the mask initially, but within a very short time they forget it's on. When we're done with the procedure, we switch the patient over to pure oxygen through the mask. *Please note though that those with COPD (chronic obstructive pulmonary disease) or those who are or think they may be pregnant shouldn't use nitrous oxide.*

ANTI-ANXIETY MEDICATIONS

Very often, a dentist will prescribe medication to allay the anxiety that can overwhelm fearful patients at the dentist. Valium is a common drug that is used for this purpose. Another good medication for anxiety with which many people are familiar is Xanax.

Xanax is the brand name for the drug alprazolam; it's most often prescribed to treat panic or anxiety disorders. Usually, if the patient hasn't had any previous experience with the drug, I'll give them a small prescription and have them "practice" taking it at home when they're not responsible for children or planning on driving. I tell them the dose to try, then see how they feel. If they feel relaxed or maybe a little sleepy, they can use that dosage for their appointment. Different people need differing levels of the medication. It depends on what other drugs they're metabolizing, and also on their disposition. The downside of this otherwise very safe drug is that it's slow to work, and slow to wear off. If patients take it too soon, they'll have to take another dose when they come in. That's why I want them to practice at home, because it takes an hour or so to reach its peak effect. Personally, I don't find Valium to be a particularly useful anti-anxiety drug—though it can help a nervous patient to sleep well the night before an appointment. It is slow to take effect and lasts a prolonged amount of time.

If you're currently taking any kind of sleeping pill, anti-anxiety drug, or anything along those lines, it's vital to let your dentist know about it, because that may react badly with the drugs you'll get at the office. Alternatively, let them know if you're already taking Xanax, because it's likely that you have some tolerance built up to the drug already, and may need a larger-than-usual dose.

ORAL SEDATION

For patients whose anxiety is not helped by the use of nitrous oxide or medications alone, there is oral sedation. This type of dentistry uses medications to aid patients to feel relaxed during their dental appointments. In most cases, the medication is a tiny pill that you take prior to your appointment with the dentist. The pill allows for moderate sedation, which means that even though you are awake and able to respond and talk, your anxiety is effectively switched off. If during the procedure more medication is needed, the dentist will administer more to make sure that you do not feel anxious. Sometimes, nitrous oxide is also used during this appointment as it assists the oral sedative in achieving the relaxation level that the patient needs. Most often the patients will not even remember the visit. Many patients say that they felt the appointment only took a few minutes, when it actually took two hours. For the severely anxious patient, oral sedation is most successful.

When a patient receives oral sedation, they will need another person to drive them to and from the appointment, and to be with them for a period of time when they return home. For most sedations, the class of drugs used are called benzodiazepines. Examples of these are Valium (diazepam), Halcion (triazolam) and Ativan (lorazepam). Usually, we use triazolam because it has a rapid onset, a predictable length of action, and a rapid elimination after its work is done. The administration of these for oral sedation should only be done by dentists who have advanced training and state licensing for the procedure. Dr. Murphy and I have such accreditations. Unfortunately, some patients with breathing health issues, such as smokers, patients with COPD or asthma, or sleep apnea, may not be candidates for oral sedation. They may, however, be able to have IV sedation.

Some people may be fearful of taking sedatives, for various reasons. Claustrophobics may find the nose mask alarming, though that's pretty rare. Other folks, especially those who have had bad experiences with dentists who crossed serious ethical boundaries, may be afraid that the drugs will stop them from being in control of what happens, and they can't deal with that. Recently, a patient told me that she was afraid to be sedated because when she was a child, a dentist had touched her inappropriately when she was in the chair, and she was terrified it would happen again. Sadly, that wasn't the first time I had heard a story like that. That's an awful thing, and I'm awed by the courage it must take for someone like her to put herself in the care of a dentist after an experience like that. In our office, a dental assistant is always present with the doctor.

I told her, "You have absolute power to control this appointment. If you have to go to the bathroom or you suddenly need a drink of water or you're just feeling overwhelmed, I will stop. I'm not going get mad at you. You don't have to be in pain, and you don't have to be scared. You are in charge. You can stop any time you want." And that goes a long way. Very few patients, after you've demonstrated that they are in control, will remain anxious.

IV SEDATION

With IV sedation, the dentist will be able to administer sedative drugs intravenously. The use of the IV means that the medications can be more accurately dosed so that a deeper level of sedation can be achieved. The patient is certainly asleep in appearance but can still respond to certain stimulations. While IV sedation has more risks than oral sedation, the incidence of complications is extremely rare. Thousands of IV sedations take place daily with great success.

LET'S TALK ABOUT DRUG INTERACTIONS FOR A MOMENT

As long as we're on the topic of medications, let's take a moment to discuss a couple of issues that people occasionally come in with—and that we really, really need to know about, because the drugs you're prescribed for one condition can cause serious problems when mixed with some of these sedatives, or by the dental work itself.

In that latter category are the phosphate drugs that some people take for osteoporosis, which is fairly common in older women, less so in men. A little-discussed but very dangerous side effect these drugs can have is that if you have a tooth extraction, which exposes bone, that area will not initiate the normal healing process and the bone in your jaw will actually become necrotic; in other words, it will die. That is not easy to stop, and can cause awful damage if it goes unchecked.

Blood thinners, too, are something we need to know about, because they increase bleeding and that can be a problem if we're doing a procedure that will cause any bleeding. If you have high blood pressure, please let your dentist know; you should not have any extractions until you've had your blood pressure checked and you're taking your medications.

> You need never go without some level of sedation if you want and need it.

WITH ALL OF THE GOOD OPTIONS AVAILABLE

You need never go without some level of sedation if you want and need it. Every chair in our office is equipped with nitrous oxide, and we're happy to supply it or any of the other drugs I've discussed. Whatever we can do to make you comfortable, we will do happily.

CHAPTER 7

Advances in Esthetic Dentistry

Dr. Scott Billings

Often during our initial consultation, new patients will tell me, "I just hate the way my teeth look!" In fact, that's frequently what finally brings them into the office, because they're working with the public or want to start dating, for instance, and they don't like what they see when they look in the mirror. Are you one of those people who wince when you catch sight of your smile? You don't have to be. Whether you're a regular visitor to your dentist's office or you've been avoiding those appointments, you may not be aware of all of the terrific improvements in dental technology that have happened in the last few years. Dentistry enjoys a robust research community, and we're constantly seeing the introduction of faster, more comfortable, and more effective means to give you the smile you've always dreamed of, but perhaps didn't think was possible.

How big a difference can esthetics make in your life? Let me put it this way: Have you ever had a day where you had your hair done just right, or you bought a dress or an outfit that made you feel like a million bucks? You know how great that feels. When you have your smile renewed, you're going to feel that way every day. You're not going to feel embarrassed; you're going to feel more confident. And if you didn't want to smile before, you're going to love smiling now.

WHITENING

Let's start with one of the simplest and most requested procedures we have available—whitening. Whitening has been around for a long time, but like so many things, has gotten much easier and quicker. Remember when only movie stars and newscasters had those super-white smiles? Today, whitening is within the reach of almost anyone, and has nearly become the new norm, esthetically, especially for people who are in public-facing jobs. It makes a huge difference in appearance, and shaves years off of your looks; in fact, research shows that others reliably judge photos of people with whiter, brighter teeth as looking younger in appearance than the same photo of the person with yellowed teeth.

We offer two kinds of whitening, and which you choose depends on your preferences and what you're looking to achieve. The first kind of whitening is done chair side; I personally prefer it because it's less likely to cause sensitivity. It also produces faster and more predictable results—and you don't have to do anything to maintain those results other than to occasionally refresh it at home. Basically, you come to the office, we paint the whitening solution onto your teeth, and then we activate it with a special light. You relax, maybe watch a little TV—and in one hour, your teeth are beautifully white. People are delighted with the results and amazed at how easy it is. Instant gratification.

In the second whitening process, tray-whitening, we create take-home trays for you that are formed to fit your teeth, both upper and lower. You put whitening gel into these, and wear them either when you sleep or for several hours daily, for about seven days. You'll touch up periodically after that. The down side is the time it takes compared to in-office whitening, and that some people report increased sensitivity.

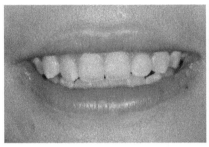
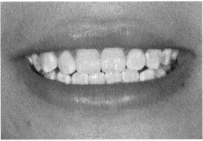

BEFORE AFTER

VENEERS

Veneers are another great way to improve the appearance of your teeth. They're exactly what they sound like; a thin layer of porcelain goes over and bonds to the front of your tooth. When we do veneers, we can change the color of the teeth and make them look whiter, and we can also change their shape. If you have spaces between your teeth, we can close those up. If you've got chipped teeth, we can make them look perfect. Even if you have a rotated tooth, meaning one that's not in line, we can change the tooth and make it look like it's in perfect alignment. I often compare the ease and effectiveness of veneers to those press-on nails women get in nail salons; they make a transformative difference in appearance but are relatively easy to do. And, of course, tooth veneers last a lot longer than press-on nails. Modern veneers are much sturdier than the early versions, lasting anywhere from ten years to a lifetime. I have some that are thirty years old and still going strong.

The veneer is applied to the tooth in a process called *dental bonding*. We begin by applying a conditioning agent to the tooth that roughens up the surface a little. Then we apply a special bonding cement, and finally the veneer itself. The process is much less invasive and quicker than doing a crown, and the results are amazing. I recently did a makeover for a young lady whose teeth went every which direction; now, with veneers on her front teeth, her smile is transformed.

> How much difference can veneers make in your appearance? The phrase "night and day" comes to mind, because it really is that dramatic.

How much difference can veneers make in your appearance? The phrase "night and day" comes to mind, because it really is that dramatic. One patient who I treated was a really nice woman who did a lot of volunteer work but had never done too much for herself. Once she got her veneers, her smile looked fantastic, and the confidence boost they provided kick-started a makeover effort for her. She started going to the gym, she got Botox, she changed her hairdo—she even got contacts. She went from matronly to "Wow!" and it all started with that great new smile.

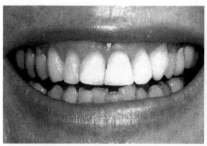 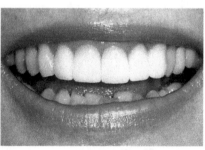

BEFORE   AFTER

COSMETIC CROWNS

A cosmetic crown covers more of the tooth than a veneer, which means the dentist has more control over the aesthetic changes that he can make and the final result. Also, today's new crowns do not have any metal, eliminating that black line we used to see at the bottom of a crown. They aren't covered with porcelain, which made old-style crowns apt to fracture. They have more of the natural translucency that tooth enamel has and look just like real teeth. They also hold up much better than older porcelain crowns did, and don't get stained or yellowed. If you've got older crowns that look dull or stained, you'll be delighted with the natural appearance we can give you with these improved crowns. If you want straighter teeth in front but you don't want to invest the money or time in braces, crowns provide a quick and long-lasting solution.

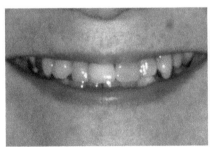 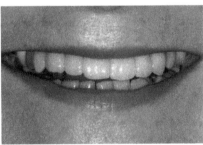

BEFORE   AFTER

INVISALIGN

Do your crooked or protruding teeth embarrass you, but you don't want to go through years of having a mouth full of braces to correct them? Invisalign is the alternative to braces that nobody will even know you're wearing. These are clear plastic aligner trays custom made by your dentist that fit onto your teeth, applying gentle, steady orthodontic force that moves them into place. Over a period of between nine and fourteen months, you are given a series of trays, which you change every two weeks until your teeth are straight. There are no wires, and no sense of pressure, so they're very comfortable. And you take them out when you eat or to clean your teeth, so there are no issues around diet restrictions or complex cleaning rituals to go through. Even if you've been told in the past that you weren't a good candidate for aligners, the technology has improved exponentially, and many people who couldn't have been successfully treated even five years ago can be treated now. Many of our Invisalign patients are women who are fifty years old and up; they tell us, "I took care of my kids first, and now I'm doing something for myself." But men and younger women are using them too and love the convenience and comfort they offer.

GINGIVECTOMY

Do you have a gummy smile? Some people's gums are too full and cover the tops of their front teeth, making them look too small for their mouths. We can fix that with what's called a gingivectomy, in which we shape and reduce the excess gum above the tooth, making the teeth look much bigger.

FIXED BRIDGEWORK

Maybe you've avoided coming to the dentist for so long that what teeth you have left are rotten or broken. But you don't want old-fashioned removable dentures, and long for more natural-looking and natural-feeling teeth. A new process allows us to effectively restore your teeth in just one day. We can make fixed bridgework attached to dental implants that will look and function like natural teeth. Best of all, it can be done in one visit: The removal of the teeth and the replacement of the bridgework can all be done in a single day, so the patient does not go without teeth at all.

Dentures are no fun for anyone—not even your dentist—because they move around, creating sore spots on your gums. But with these new implant-supported hybrid dentures, what you're chewing on is connected to your jaw, just like your teeth, so there's no movement. It's really like getting your teeth back. We design your new smile using a digital scan, and we can build you a set of teeth that will rival what you had. In fact, if you didn't like the teeth you had, we can make you look even better.

> We design your new smile using a digital scan, and we can build you a set of teeth that will rival what you had.

It's worth noting that if you're a fearful patient, all of this work can be done while you're sedated—and the actual procedure can be done in a single day.

DENTAL IMPLANTS

Dental implants have made a huge difference in how we do dentistry, because now we can actually offer people the chance to recover the ability to chew, to maintain the health of their mouth, or to replace dentures with functional and attractive teeth that stay in place. What used to be a very complex and specialized process is now routinely taught in dental school, so you don't have to go to a specialist to get an implant any more. They used to be much more expensive, too, and not nearly as well made or as attractive and functional as they are now. We can put an implant in nearly anyone's mouth and in nearly any position, and the process is much safer and simpler, too.

DERMAL FILLERS AND BOTOX

Something you may not have thought of in terms of esthetic treatments a dentist would offer is Botox and other dermal fillers. Why would injectables be offered by a dentist? Well, for one thing, nobody is more adept than a dentist when it comes to injections—and nobody knows more about the structures of your mouth and face than your dentist does.

Age and tooth loss can create or deepen lines around the mouth that make us look older. Lips, too, tend to become thinner and less full as we age, and this, too, can be successfully treated with dermal fillers. Those harsh lines between your eyebrows and the crows' feet beside the eyes can also be erased. If you're getting your smile refreshed, it's a great way to make your appearance that much more youthful.

> Everyone wants to look their best—and as dentistry has advanced, the kinds of esthetic remedies we can offer you have gotten better and easier, too.

Everyone wants to look their best—and as dentistry has advanced, the kinds of esthetic remedies we can offer you have gotten better and easier, too. If you've spent too many years hiding your smile because of missing, misshapen, discolored, or out-of-alignment teeth, please call us for a consultation. We can talk you through the possibilities and get you the treatment you need to have a smile you'll be proud to show the world.

CHAPTER 8

Choosing Your Dentist

Dr. Scott Billings

Choosing the right dentist is just as important to your health and well-being as choosing your medical doctor. In both instances, it's critical to your wellness that you find someone who makes you feel comfortable and whom you can trust. That's because ideally these will be long-term relationships, and your ability to relate to your practitioner will impact how willing you are to go in for treatment when you need it, how honest you're likely to be with them, and whether you're confident in accepting their recommendations.

Of course, the first thing you'll want to know will probably be about their background; where they went to school, and how long they have been in practice, for instance. All of that information should be available on their website, and you should be able to get a clear picture there, too, of the kinds of services they offer.

It's likely that in this Google-centric age that some of your research will be done online, and that's a very good place to begin reviewing how other patients feel about the dentist you're considering. Google reviews can tell you a lot: did the patient writing the review feel good about the experience they had? Is the doctor described as patient, caring, and kind? Did the doctor spend time talking with the patient, or were they rushed through their appointment? Were they kept waiting, or taken into their appointment on time? What kinds of amenities does the reviewer describe, in terms of comforts offered? Were they happy with the work they had done? People writing reviews online tend to be very frank about both the good points and the bad, so that's a good way to do deeper research after you've had a look at the dentist's website.

Did a friend recommend a dentist to you? If that person also has issues with dental anxiety, their reference is useful. If they don't have much to say about the dental practice other than, "Well, we always go to them," though, that may be more a reflection of their disinclination to make a change than anything else.

But if you suffer from dental fears or anxiety, making the right choice is especially important, because you're far less likely to go to a dentist than most people are, even when you need one—and having the wrong one—someone who makes you feel uncomfortable, not understood, or unwelcome—will make you more inclined than ever to avoid going in for the treatment you need. If someone's a grouch, displays impatience, or make you feel disrespected, how likely are you to want to see them? Not very likely!

TAKE CHARGE!

That's why, when you're looking for a dentist, it's much smarter to be proactive, not reactive. It may have been a very long time since you had a regular office visit or a cleaning. Don't wait for an emergency to come up before finding a practitioner you can feel comfortable with, because when you're already in pain and feeling fearful, you're not going to be happy having to go to a stranger—but you'll have to, if you haven't established a relationship with a dentist you can trust.

Whether you're looking to find an alternative to your current practitioner, or ready to find a new practitioner after having gone without one for a long while, put yourself in the driver's seat, and realize that *you're* in charge. You're the consumer, and you have choices. If

> When you're looking for a dentist, it's much smarter to be proactive, not reactive.

you're a fearful patient, then you want to make sure that the practice you choose is especially good at working with people with those kinds of issues. Here are some ideas for how you can find that "best fit" practice when you're shopping for a new dentist.

REQUEST A CONSULTATION-ONLY APPOINTMENT

Many of our potential patients request an initial non-clinical appointment, to meet us and to look around. They don't want the examination, they just want to check us out. We welcome that kind of "getting to know you" visit, and encourage them to come in. Don't be embarrassed to tell the person who answers your call at the practice, "I'm a fearful patient, and I need a doctor that I'm going to be comfortable with, and to be able to trust. Can I come in for a consultation just to meet the doctor?" Some doctors simply won't do that, even for an anxious patient—and that's fine, because you don't want to work with that doctor anyway.

The answer to that question should be, "Yes, that's not a problem. We understand your anxiety and we'd be delighted to meet you and show you around." You're off to a great start if you get an answer along those lines, because that shows they're tuned in to your needs and are willing to make time to accommodate you. If they try to push you into scheduling an exam during that call, even if you've made it clear you don't want that, that says something about the practice that you're not going to like, because they're putting their needs ahead of yours. Maybe their first priority isn't you as a patient. You shouldn't have to commit to any kind of exam, much less a cleaning or other treatment, to be able to sit down with a prospective dentist.

We typically book a twenty-minute consultation with any new patient who asks for one. That gives us time to sit down and discuss the patient's needs, their fears, and what we can do to help them. There's no pressure, nor should there be.

Some patients feel safe enough to go ahead and book an exam in that initial visit—but that's really all that any practice should do the first time they see you. In dentistry, the way it's nearly always been done is that when you go to a new dentist, they first do x-rays, then they're going to start you out by cleaning your teeth, and only after that will the dentist do an exam. We never do that; if a patient is comfortable with getting an exam, then we always start there, because we don't believe in recommending any kind of treatment before we know exactly what your needs are—not even a cleaning. Why? Because we don't know until we've examined you just what kind of cleaning you need—and yes, there is more than one kind of cleaning. In our practice, you'll get a comprehensive exam first, and you and the dentist will go over all of the findings from that exam so that you're clear on what treatments might be recommended and why. Sometimes, a standard cleaning isn't what you need, and we believe that an educated patient is equipped to make the best choices.

BE HONEST ABOUT YOUR FEARS

If you're an anxious patient, your dentist needs to be more than a great clinician. They need to be someone who listens, who's compassionate, and who understands dental anxiety and will work with you. They have to be as willing to address your fears as they are to treat your oral conditions. If they're pushing you to come in for the standard cleaning and exam at that first visit, then they're not addressing your anxiety needs, they're just dumping you into the hygienist's lap.

When I meet with an anxious patient, we don't even talk about their teeth at first. I start by listening to them: what are they fearful about, what have their experiences been, and how are they feeling? I validate their feelings and let them know that I understand, and that no matter what their experiences have been in the past, they're safe here; that I know they don't want to have these feelings, but that they can't help it, and that those feelings will be respected.

Then, I explain what I can do to help them get past their anxiety, so they can get the help they want and need. What I try to do in having this conversation is to leave them feeling hopeful, knowing that someone understands, empathizes, and has the means and the desire to help them. More than once I've had patients who burst into tears, telling me, "No dentist ever talked to me like that before!"

DON'T COVER UP OR SHRUG OFF YOUR FEARS

So often, people are embarrassed to talk about their anxieties with a prospective dentist, often because others have scoffed at them or tried to shame them out of their fears. But please, when you're interviewing a dentist, don't let shame keep you from being forthright about your issues. Otherwise, you will fall back into the trap where your anxiety is stronger than the dentist's ability to help you to deal with it, and you're going stop your treatment as you've probably always done in the past. If you feel dismissed, unheard, or otherwise disrespected, find another dentist.

Your experience begins with how your call is handled by the person running the front desk. Ask questions and be direct: "What methods does your dentist use to help fearful patients receive treatment without feeling so anxious?" Listen to the answer—not just what is said, but how it's said. If the answer is vague, like, "Oh well, he's got things he does …" or if they're dismissive, "Don't worry about it, he's used to nervous patients"—you might want to try another office. If you get a solid answer, such as, "Our doctor treats many anxious patients, and they learn a lot about their anxiety. It's important to our doctor to help them get their treatment and help them do it in a way where they're not as anxious. And yes, we treat a lot … " That person is an ambassador to anxious patients, and that tells you where the heart of the practice is. "We'll take you under our wing and help you," or some version of that reassurance is what you want to hear.

When you come in to meet with the dentist initially, you will have to gauge that person's demeanor and attitude. Are they truly excited about helping an anxious patient, or are they shrugging off your anxiety, with phrases like, "Don't worry about that. We'll make sure you don't feel anything." If they say things like that, it's a big tip-off. But if you go in and you come out of the initial meeting feeling warm and fuzzy—even though you're an anxious patient—you have probably found the right dentist.

I mentioned earlier that working with a dentist is ideally a long-term relationship. It's also a deeply personal one—intimate, even, in the sense that you're in the position of trusting this person to work inside your mouth while you're lying down in a chair, with your mouth open and your head back. You're counting on this person to be careful, caring, and gentle, and you're quite literally in his or her hands. Once you have someone you trust in that space, it's hard to consider going to someone else. That's especially true for the anxious patient, because trust issues play a big part in that. Is this someone who might be cavalier about causing you pain? Or is this a person who you know is going to be extra careful not to hurt you?

So, one of the first questions you'll want to ask your prospective dentist is, "Are you comfortable working with someone who doesn't want to be here?" The answer to that should be along the lines of, "A lot of people feel that way and we've been able to help them," rather than, "Don't worry about that." Ask the dentist, "Are you willing to stop what you're doing whenever I ask you to?" Ideally, the answer should be, "Yes, of course—always," and followed with some questions from the dentist to you, about what typically makes you anxious and when you've asked dentists to stop what they were doing in the past.

Whatever the wording, the overriding message you hear should be, "We're here to help you. We want to be the special practice that makes you able to get your treatment done and not feel anxious." Upbeat, positive, reassuring, validating— that's what they should be, not someone who's switching the topic or brushing you off.

> If you feel the scales tipping toward hope and acceptance, listen to those feelings, because this is very likely the dentist you need.

Part of making this decision is emotional, too, and you need to be prepared for the fact that your anxiety emotions are going to fight with your acceptance emotions—the sense that, "I feel like with this dentist I can do this." If you feel the scales tipping toward hope and acceptance, listen to those feelings, because this is very likely the dentist you need.

DON'T BE ASHAMED

Some patients who've avoided seeing a dentist for a long time feel ashamed of how their teeth look. If the dentist doing the initial exam makes those feelings worse by saying things like, "We've got to get in there," or, "What took you so long to get in here?" or even, "Oh, wow, what a mess!" that clearly shows a lack of sensitivity and caring. Nobody needs to be berated for not having cared for their teeth, and the anxious patient needs that least of all. You know you need help—that's why you've come in. That's something to be proud of, and any practitioner who makes you feel worse about your teeth is not the person for you.

The thing is, there are always different and more caring ways to express uncomfortable facts. Where one practitioner might say, "This tooth is bombed out, it's got to go," to me that's unnecessarily negative and not the best way to describe a badly decayed tooth to an anxious patient. My choice of words would be a little more clinical and more upbeat: "Unfortunately we're not going to be able to save that tooth, but we can take care of it," is a lot more reassuring.

But, please, don't let shame or embarrassment prevent you from seeing a dentist. If they make you feel badly about it, find another one. There are plenty of good, caring people out there, and doing your research should help you find someone you can be comfortable with.

FIND A PRACTICE THAT OFFERS
MULTIPLE SERVICES

Let's say you've found a practice that you really like—one where you feel safe, respected, and comfortable. But one day, your favorite dentist tells you that you need some special treatment—perhaps an implant or a root canal, for instance—that their practice doesn't offer. Now, you're being given a referral to another practice and another dentist or specialist—someone you have never even met. The dentist you've been referred to may be very good and entirely trustworthy—but, unfortunately, trust isn't transferrable, so you may find yourself hesitating to follow through with the treatment your dentist wants you to have, because you don't want to go through the process of learning to trust this new person. That puts you back to square one.

That's why it's important to ask about treatments or procedures beyond the usual fillings and crown when you initially speak to your perspective dentist. Do they refer the more-complex treatments out, or do they have the expertise to do them in-house? For most people, that's just a matter of convenience, but for a fearful patient, it can be tremendously reassuring to know that your dentist can handle most everything you'll need without having to refer you out to another practitioner.

In our practice, we're constantly expanding our skills, our technologies, and our services, because we have patients who tell us, "I won't go to anyone but you," and we want to be able to serve them. We do implants, root canals, and many other complex procedures on a regular basis, because we want our patients to get the care they need right here.

The more you know going into an office, the better you're going to feel about working with the dentist. Knowledge is power and putting the power of choice into your hands is why it's a good idea to find a dentist you like and feel comfortable with before some dental emergency leaves you in pain and distress, thumbing through the phone book or desperately searching the internet. Do your homework ahead of time; find someone you like, in a practice that makes you feel welcome, and you'll feel much better knowing you've found a practice that is right for you, and someone you can call if something goes wrong.

"WHAT SHOULD I EXPECT AT MY FIRST APPOINTMENT?"

Your positive experience should start when you make that first phone call to a potential practice. The person who answers the phone should be cheerful, pleasant, and informative. If you have questions about the practice, that person should be able to answer them, and not trying to rush you off the phone.

> Your positive experience should start when you make that first phone call to a potential practice.

When you first call Eastern Shore Dental Care, we'll ask how you heard about us. We'll get some contact information from you, and then reserve your first appointment. When you walk through the door for the first time, we want you to feel at home. We start with an office tour, which includes the background and history of the practice and information on the training and experience of our doctors.

We know that for many people, simply getting themselves to make that first call is a big personal victory. That's why we offer free initial consultation appointments to anyone who wants to meet us, because we know how tough it is for the phobic person to even come into the office, never mind having an exam from a stranger. Any dentist who treats phobic patients ought to offer those, and if the person making your appointment says they don't do that, you'll probably need to keep shopping. If they do offer them, go in and see what they're all about.

Alternatively, you might feel comfortable enough to say, "I'd like to have the examination, but I don't want to schedule hygiene work until I have an examination, please. Can I do that?" If they tell you that new patients always have to see the hygienist, feel free to tell them goodbye.

When you arrive for your first visit at the practice, the person at the desk should greet you in a friendly and welcoming way. You should be given a tour of the offices, including a look at a treatment room, and be able to find out what kinds of treatments they do there. Are they a full-service office, or do they typically send patients to specialists for certain kinds of procedures, such as root canals? What kinds of amenities do they have to offer, in terms of comfort? Are there noise-cancelling headphones available for your use? Do they offer you nitrous oxide if you want it, without making an issue out of it? All your general questions about the practice should be answered fully and without hesitation.

Finally, your prospective dentist should take the time to sit down with you and get to know you a little bit. We always have a nice general chat with new patients who are considering our practice and try to learn not only about their dental needs, but also about who they are as individuals. We encourage them to open up about their fears, if that's a problem for them, and work to reassure them. Hopefully, the dentist already knows that you're a fearful patient, because the person who made your appointment initially has told him or her. But don't hesitate to bring that up, because this appointment is about you, and you're doing your due diligence. Talk frankly about your feelings and pay attention to how engaged the dentist is in really listening to you. If they look like they're checking their watch or just waiting for you to stop talking, then that may signal a certain disinterest in your issues. You can tell, too, if they're genuinely responding to your needs and what you're asking for. Your gut is probably your best indicator for how you'll feel with this person, which is why it matters that they're willing to take time with you. It's not about whether they sound smart or not, it's about likability: "He/she gets me, and I feel comfortable."

Ask the practitioner specifically what they do to help nervous patients get through a procedure. Will they dependably stop what they're doing if you raise your hand? We're here to treat patients, and not all patients are the same. And if a patient needs a break, to stop for a moment to swallow, to spit, just to catch their breath, or to go to the restroom, then of course we let them. Any other answer than that is unacceptable. If you find yourself overwhelmed and can't finish a procedure, are they willing to stop for the day and let you come back? Someone whose answer suggests they're a busy practice and run on a tight schedule is probably not the dentist for you.

Do they have a track record of success with fearful patients, and can they share some of those stories with you? Get in front of that dentist and be ready to gauge your emotion. If you're uncomfortable with him, if you don't feel that positivity, then maybe, as an emotional patient, you're setting yourself up for another failure with another dentist who just isn't the right person for you. And you should hold out for somebody who gives you that emotional positivity, so you will then be able to keep growing your success in beating the anxiety that's stopping you from getting treatment. If you know you're going to want sedation, ask about that at your initial consultation; what do they offer in the office to help you through a procedure? If you have problems with gagging or claustrophobia, ask if they use a 3-D scanner rather than old-fashioned impressions, because that's going to be a much more comfortable experience for you.

> Nothing is more gratifying to us than hearing from our patients, "You got me over my anxiety!"

Nothing is more gratifying to us than hearing from our patients, "You got me over my anxiety!" One patient was so anxious when she began that she simply could not make herself come back, even though she knew she needed treatment. My dental assistant, who's a wonderful ally for our anxious patients, would call her periodically just to reassure her, and help build her confidence up in herself and the practice. She'd say, "We'll get through this—you can do it, and we can help you." Finally, the woman was able to come in and get the work she needed done. It took a lot of handholding and a lot of nitrous, but she's feeling great about herself and her new smile. Now, she comes in and laughs about how nervous she used to be.

I think often, too, of the formerly anxious patient who told me how proud she was that she could smile now like other people, with her lips open instead of keeping them clamped closed to hide her teeth. She told me it had changed her life, and I could see she meant it.

We see the same patients for years, because once they've worked with us, they just won't go anywhere else. And most satisfying of all is that so many of them who started out needing a lot of reassurance or sedation, for instance, no longer do. Sometimes they tell us, "I'm not afraid at all anymore." That's so meaningful, especially when we look at where they were when they came to us initially: so anxious, often in pain, and showing the effects of years of neglect of their oral health.

That's what you have to look forward to, and why it's worth it to make that difficult first phone call and get the process started. It's a great pot of gold at the end of the rainbow for you, when you're able to achieve being able to go to the dentist, not having to worry about your fear anymore, and to have healthy teeth and a beautiful smile. It brings you self-confidence and self-actualization. It lets you feel good about yourself, because you did something positive and you have results to show for it.

We like to think we go above and beyond in welcoming potential patients, and in making them comfortable once they're here. From the moment you step into Eastern Shore Dental Care, we want you to feel comfortable and relaxed. We want to get to know you so we can best serve those needs, so we strive to make each new patient experience a special one. We even give you a nice gift, too, to welcome you. For us, it's another way to show you that we're patient centered, and that you matter.

Pick your own music once seated. Select a warm back massage in one of our state-of-the-art chairs. TVs mounted to the ceilings will keep your mind off of the treatment. We offer free Wi-Fi. Let us treat you to a cup of coffee from the Keurig or a cold bottle of water. Feel free to request an iPod, blanket, lip balm, or any number of items from our Comfort Menu, designed to put you at ease.

In Closing

When we met Robbie, he was thirty-five years old and he'd had a rough life. The son of a drug addict, he'd done some work for us at the office as a handyman, and it was one of our hygienists who asked us if we'd look at his teeth. He wanted to get married, but his girlfriend had told him she wouldn't marry him until he got his teeth fixed—and when we examined him, we certainly could see why. Virtually every tooth had a major problem, and most of them couldn't be fixed. Either he needed a whole mouth full of implants or a full set of dentures—and he had no money for either option. He was also afraid of dentists and of getting dental work done, but at this point, he was more afraid of losing his girlfriend.

We examined him, we talked about it, and we decided to do the work for free, and make him a whole set of dentures. When the dental assistant went into the examining room to tell Robbie the news, he burst into tears of joy. He couldn't believe this life-changing thing was going to happen.

For us, it wasn't that big a deal, in the sense of time and expense. But it was a very big deal for him—and being able to do something like this for someone like him, to change his life—that's a big deal for us, every time. We got him in the chair, sedated him, and fitted him out for his new teeth.

It's hard for many of us to imagine what it would be like to have teeth that were so awful looking that even someone who loved you just couldn't see past your appearance—but that happens, and for some of the phobic or fearful people we treat, that's the impetus that finally gets them to our offices for treatment. For others, it's a dental crisis they can no longer ignore: a broken or lost tooth, or the pain of a bad one. What they all have in common is that, once they've been treated, they're so very glad to have found us. Our patients are dedicated to us, because we're dedicated to treating them with the kindness, empathy, and respect they deserve. We really care about them—and we understand their pain. Our mission statement is framed on the wall, and it speaks to our commitment to patient care: We are committed to providing a lifetime of extraordinary service to our family of patients, and to give generously to our community. We strive to set the standard for compassion, and to exceed the expectations of those under our care.

> Our patients are dedicated to us, because we're dedicated to treating them with the kindness, empathy, and respect they deserve.

That commitment to give generously to the community is part of why we decided to help Robbie, and he isn't the only *pro bono* case we've done. Every year, we participate in a program called Smiles from the Heart. One Saturday a year, we open our office to all: first come, first served. We advertise it on the radio, the local papers, the community churches, and on social media. Patients who come that day can get a filling, a cleaning, or even an extraction for free. We see these patients one after another, all day, and usually around 120 people come through the doors. All of our staff volunteer to join us, our associate doctors help us, and we have other doctors who volunteer to come in, too. It's a long day of work, but it's the kind of work that leaves everyone feeling great about what we do. The turnout gets bigger every year as word spreads, and that's great. It gives us tremendous joy to know we're helping folks who wouldn't get help otherwise, and that we can make a real difference in someone's life and health.

That ability to change lives isn't limited to the needy; we've seen so many lives changed for the better when those who are fearful finally find the courage to call us. If you've been putting off treatment you know you need for too long because of dental fears or phobia, here's an invitation. Visit our website—www.easternshoredentalcare.com— or give us a call. Read our Google reviews—you'll be reassured by how many of our patients had anxiety, too, until they came to us. Come in for a consultation; meet us, meet the team, and see our offices. It's free, and it gives you a chance to see what we're about without any stress or expectations. It's a great first step in the right direction, and we're sure that once you've met with us, you'll feel much more comfortable about going ahead with a new patient visit and exam the next time. When we do examine you, we sit down and take time with you, discussing your results, what you need, and how it could be accomplished. Yes, that's a little unusual—but we understand that information is power, and we're committed to putting the power in your hands. In short, we treat you the way we'd want to be treated ourselves.

> We treat you the way we'd want to be treated ourselves.

And we should note too that we can do nearly any kind of work right here in our offices, including the kinds of things that dentists typically send patients to specialists to have done: implants, even root canals. Why? Because our patients don't want to have to go elsewhere to be treated; they've come to trust us, but trust isn't so easily transferred. That's why we're constantly adding to our skills and our services.

We told you earlier about the patient whose teeth were so badly worn down that she'd lost about 50 percent of her tooth structure. It took a lot of patience and time to convince her that she could trust us; her fear of dentists was why her case had gotten so bad in the first place. But, ultimately, we won her over, and wound up crowning every tooth, opening her bite, and restoring the size of her teeth. And at her last visit when we were wrapping up, she told us, "You know what? I didn't feel like I had to take my medicine. I wasn't even afraid to come in." That was someone who had been hugely afraid, and let her teeth go so badly. To hear that at the end of a lengthy treatment plan was the ultimate reward.

We hope you'll give us a call and come and meet us. You'll see the difference in your very first visit.

WHAT OUR PATIENTS SAY

"As soon as I walked into the office, I felt at ease. The staff is very friendly and compassionate. They listen to your needs and understand you. I've never been to a dentist and felt the way I do when I walk in here. Definitely would recommend to anyone that needs a dentist."

"Their new office is a Zen zone. Very calming and soothing! The doctors and hygienists are so nice and they keep you informed every step of the way. They are very gentle and friendly and concerned for your comfort."

"The best dental office you will ever find! I have been a patient of this practice for over twenty years. I receive many compliments on my teeth. Dr. Murphy and Beth are the greatest! They are very professional, and take time to check, and clean my teeth. I highly recommend going to Eastern Shore Dental Care. They offer excellent dental care plans. They treat you like family."

"Going to the dentist doesn't even feel like a doctor's visit! The staff is always extremely nice, the office is beautiful, they have great music playing. If I could give them a ten I would."

"I've been going to this practice for almost thirty years. They are so friendly and knowledgeable. The staff is so welcoming and their new office makes you feel like you are going to the spa. My husband just recently started going and he has been so happy with all of their help to repair his teeth. I wouldn't want to go anywhere else."

"The staff is so nice and caring. You get state-of-the-art treatment in a beautiful new office. It is always a pleasant experience being treated there."

"I have never loved going to the dentist until I came here. The staff is so welcoming and professional and they care about the patient. I am no longer scared to go to the dentist!"

Meet Dr. Billings and Dr. Murphy

Dr. Scott Billings

My interest in helping anxious patients and in the health field in general certainly started because of my mom, who was a medical technologist when I was a kid. She worked in a lab where she was tasked with doing blood draws and performing hematology tests and blood counts. Back in those days, the medical technologists wore a white nurse's uniform, so I would see her every day going off to the hospital in her uniform. I remember going to work to visit her as a kid and seeing the way she related to her patients. Most people aren't all that happy about getting blood work done, and some of her patients were very fearful. Mom had a great personality, very warm and genuine, and people always liked her immediately. She was wonderful at talking to her patients, calming their nerves, and getting them through their procedures. I learned a lot about dealing with nervous patients just by watching how she interacted with them, and when I went off to college, I decided that I wanted to be in the health field, too, but I wasn't sure which field to choose.

Once I got to college, I tried several different majors; my first choice was pre-veterinary science; from there, I switched to pre-medical technology, then into pharmacy, and finally, I decided that the dental field sounded interesting to me. It was a health field, and one that allowed for one-on-one relationships and contacts with patients. The dental field was unique because you get to see patients over and over for years, as opposed to other health fields, where you help them through their ailment at the time and then never see them again. I liked the idea of a continuing relationship with my patients.

I think the reason it took me nearly to my second year to choose dentistry was that I just didn't have much understanding of the field until I began to explore it. Although I went to the dentist growing up, I didn't really understand all that a dentist does. It turns out I love the job—I always have. I love the patients, and the fun we have just meeting people, and talking to them about anything and everything. We talk about their personal life and their kids. We talk about where they went on vacation and what kind of dog they have. It's a great fit for a people person.

The other part that really appealed to me is that, when I do my dental procedures, I'm usually able to complete them in one visit, which means I get to see what I've accomplished. I have that instant gratification as my reward for a job well done. In other fields, people will often work on projects with a team, over a period of years—and even so, it's often just one small part of a much larger effort. Then they pass it on to the next team, who advances it, and they never really see the results of what they did. In dentistry, you get to see the results, and there's the deep satisfaction which comes with knowing you really made a difference for your patient. You get to share the joy of making them better, with them present.

And, while my mom's great example provided a big part of my understanding of how to deal with people who were fearful, I have to say that the most memorable lesson was one I got when I was working as a student in a Baltimore dental clinic. I'd been assigned a patient to work on, in this case, a young boy who made it very clear he didn't want to be there. When I came toward him, he sprang from the chair and ran out of the treatment room, screaming like a banshee. What could I do? I had to go after him, so I did, white coat flapping. But he was faster than me and made it to the waiting room where about two hundred horrified Baltimoreans got to watch me chase him around their chairs until I finally caught up with him. A great instructor saw the ruckus and took over; he got the boy back in the chair, and he went over techniques of how to present the patient what you're about to do, how to explain it so it's not scary to them, and how to put control of what would happen into their hands. He told the boy if he was scared or something hurt, all he had to do was to raise his hand. He explained that if he were going to do anything that might be painful, like the pinch the boy might feel when he got an injection, he'd tell him about it first. It was a great lesson on how to empower even the youngest patient and allay their fears, and I've never forgotten it.

When I graduated, I knew I wanted my own practice. I had only been out of school for about three months when I found one I liked, and within a year I purchased it and started working. Luckily, I was in the right place at the right time; on Kent Island in Maryland, where there were a lot of new homes going in, and in the 1980s when I first was here, the island's population about doubled. A lot of people on the western shore, the more suburban area, were moving to the island, which was more rural, and, thanks to them, we grew rapidly.

As a young practitioner starting out, I could always tell right away when I had someone in the chair who was fearful or phobic. I put a lot of thought into how to help them, because I knew that it didn't help to be impatient with them, or to belittle them, or to rush them, and that wasn't my instinct. I learned to be ever more patient, slower, and calmer—and that helped my patients relax. Luckily for me, I have an easy-going personality, and my mom's example to follow. I noticed that there were different levels of anxiety my patients would experience, and I wanted to make sure that I was able to help. We made sure to get nitrous oxide, and that was our go-to to help some patients. Then anti-anxiety drugs became more available, so I would use some of those on patients to help them. It was met with great success, and I saw that over time, as patients learned to trust me, their anxiety would diminish to the point where it wasn't an issue for them. That was a great feeling, because I could see that some of these folks hadn't been to a dentist in a long time, and now I could help them. Knowing I could give them back their smiles, and their trust, was a terrific feeling then, and still is.

It was just a few years later that I met Dr. Murphy, and he came to work for me. In 1990, we became partners. It was a good match— we do our dentistry in the same way, and we're both committed to compassionate care for fearful patients. Thanks to more advanced sedation techniques and drugs, we are able to help even the most fearful, anxious patients.

I should probably mention that my mom also introduced me to my wife; we've been going strong for more than forty years now, so I think Mom did a pretty good job of choosing. We have four great kids; none of them are dentists, but all of them are committed to working in or discovering careers they love. Thanks, Mom!

When I'm not doing dentistry, I'm probably either out golfing, or playing my guitar and singing Beatles covers at a local open mic night with friends.

Dr. Scott Billings is a graduate of the University of Maryland School of Dentistry and founded the practice on Kent Island in 1981. In 2016, he was named Queen Anne's County Business Leader of the Year by the Chamber of Commerce. He has also received numerous other accolades, including: "Favorite Business Owner" and "Favorite Dentist" by The Shore Update, "Top Doc" and "Top Invisalign Provider" by What's Up! Eastern Shore; "Favorite Doc" by Chesapeake Family Magazine. In the fall of 2017, he and Dr. Chris Murphy were presented an official citation from Senator Steve Hershey on behalf of the Maryland General Assembly in recognition of their, "Commitment to the health and well-being of the residents of the Eastern Shore." He has been featured on local TV and radio stations all over the Eastern Shore, including WBOC-TV (Salisbury), WCTR 96.1 (Chestertown), and WCEI 96.7 (Easton.) Dr. Billings is married and has four adult children. He has advanced training in cosmetic and implant dentistry and enjoys creating beautiful smile makeovers.

Dr. Chris Murphy

When people ask what made me so committed to compassionate care for fearful patients, I always tell them the story of the dentist who terrorized me when I was a kid. He'd started out working on me with the promise that he'd stop if I needed him to—but I guess I taxed his patience (such as it was) and at some point in my treatment he kept going when I told him he was hurting me, saying "Just hold still!" That made a big impression on me. First, he'd been untruthful, because he'd promised he'd stop. And second, it was clear to me that he didn't care whether he was hurting me or not. While he didn't succeed in making me phobic, he certainly set the gold standard for what *not* to do. I can tell you that as a dentist, I'd never be dishonest with a patient or fail to stop when asked to do so.

Unfortunately, they teach you some awful techniques in dental school. There's a device called the papoose board which is used on frightened children to force them into compliance. It's more like a straitjacket, in that a child is literally strapped into it to keep him from moving. As unbelievable as it seems, this thing is still used by some dentists. That's not something I'd ever use, and I think that any dentist who would isn't putting the patient's welfare first. I think they're thinking of their own welfare, their desire to get the job done and to move on, and that makes them impatient. If you can't summon up any compassion for a scared child, you might not belong in dentistry—or anywhere in health care, frankly. It's so much better to take the time with the patient and explain what you're doing; to ask for feedback, and to reassure them. That approach works, and it's the one I'm comfortable with.

I came to the health care field mostly because I was good at science; I was good at chemistry, so I started out as a chemistry major in college. Looking around at the career possibilities, I could see that there were a lot of great opportunities in the health care field, and that the classes that were prerequisites were all things that I like to do, and I did well at. My dad was an aeronautical engineer, and I think he'd hoped I'd follow him into engineering, but I had my own path.

I think what ultimately made me want to do dentistry rather than medicine was the certainty that dentistry offers that you're doing the right thing for your patient. Diagnosing a dental issue is relatively easy, whereas diagnosing a patient as a doctor is tough, and so much is at stake. In dentistry, we can reliably spot the problem and cure our patients—and that's not always the case in medicine. I know I'd have found it very unsatisfactory to spend my career wondering if I'd made the right call or worrying about treating a patient properly. In dentistry, it's easy to see what's wrong or right, and that knowledge that you're doing the right thing for your patient is very satisfying. And I love the long-term relationships and interactions with my patients. I think, in general, I'm a people person, but I was stunned by how much I enjoy that part of it. While I still enjoy the technical aspects of the work, what really is rewarding is working with people and earning their trust.

I have a lot of patients who will only come in when I'm available, because they trust me and they don't want anyone else to work on them. That's a huge ego boost, and it's a reward that you don't get in many occupations. In other professions, you might be recognized for your work by your peers or colleagues, but having patients put so much trust in you is really humbling and meaningful to me. I just love it when people say, "You better not quit, because I'm never going to go to anybody else." When I decided that I wanted to go to dental school, that kind of patient love and trust was a blessing than I never expected. I anticipated doing all the work of dentistry, but I didn't know how much their caring would mean to me. I'm just doing mechanical things, in the kindest way I can, the easiest way I can. I've been practicing for thirty-two years, and I still look forward to getting to work and seeing my patients. I love getting kids or adults to trust me and relax. It's such worthwhile work, and I know I'm helping them on so many levels. Working with Dr. Billings is great, because we both feel the same way about this, and we're always comparing notes on what helps our patients.

I think dentists in general get confrontational needlessly with kids. I remember the day when a little kid came in for a filling but was too scared to get into the chair. Instead of sending him home or having his mother hold him down (yes, some dentists do that, too), I just started showing him all the equipment. I took a low-speed hand piece and ran it lightly over his thumbnail; because the nail is like a tooth, I could show him that it's a similar feeling. If you vibrate someone's tooth and they're not expecting that sensation, it can panic them. However, if you do that on their nail, and they get an idea of what it's going to feel like, then suddenly it's a lot less threatening to let me put it on a tooth. When I see they're taking that in, I always ask permission before moving forward.

When I'm giving an injection, I just tell the child that it's going to pinch. If they ask me if it's a needle, I say, "Well, it's pokey." I don't lie to them. I explain that I'm going to give their tooth a little sleepy juice. Then I'll say, "Close your eyes," and we'll just get on with it. Sometimes it pinches, and sometimes it doesn't, so I'll ask them, while I'm injecting them, "Did you feel the pinches?" Some of them will say no, and then I'll say, "Great, then you probably won't feel it at all." If they do feel the pinch, I say, "Did you feel the pinch?" And they're happy to tell me, "Yeah, I did feel the pinch." But they're not scared, because I was honest with them up front, and they knew what to expect. They know the pinch is going to go away, and the whole time I'm injecting them, slowly. Most of us are a lot more comfortable in challenging circumstances if we know what to expect, and kids are no different. Being forthright with them is a way to show them respect, and they respond with trust. Sometimes after a shot, a child will get fearful when the numbness kicks in—"I feel like my lips are falling off." I hand them a mirror so they can see they look normal, and they calm down.

I always tell my patients to raise their hand if they need me to stop for any reason, and unlike my old dentist, I always do stop. If it's a child, I tell them, "Good job, you raised your hand!" because I want them to know I'm glad they're communicating with me. Then they're likely to feel, "Okay, I can trust this guy."

I have two grownup kids: my daughter is an occupational therapy technician, and my son is a lawyer. I'm still trying to figure out what my "keeper" hobby is; I keep trying new ones, then moving on, but so far, I've run six marathons, done a lot of long-distance bike riding, and taken several biking trips across the Rockies. I also got my pilot's license and was enjoying flying planes until I had the interesting experience of semi-crash-landing a small plane when its landing gear broke off. That cured me of piloting. I still ski every year, and love to travel with my wife. Lately, I'm enjoying driving fast cars quite a bit, and Dr. Billings's trying to talk me into racing my car at a track.

Dr. Chris Murphy partnered with Dr. Scott Billings in 1986. He is a graduate of the University of Maryland School of Dentistry and completed postgraduate education studies for implant restorations and cosmetic dentistry. Dr. Murphy was prominently featured in the May 2017 issue of Dental Town Magazine—a national industry-leading publication—for his mission work performed around the world. He has also been widely recognized in the area as the following: "Favorite Business

Owner" and "Favorite Dentist" by readers of The Shore Update; "Top Doc" and "Top Invisalign Provider" by readers of "What's Up! Eastern Shore; "Favorite Doc" by readers of Chesapeake Family Magazine. In the fall of 2017, Dr. Murphy was recognized by the Maryland General Assembly for his work in the community.

Contact Us

EASTERN SHORE DENTAL CARE

22 Kent Towne Market
Chester, MD 21619

New Patients: 443-249-8881
Current Patients: 443-249-8854
Fax: 410-643-8538

www.easternshoredentalcare.com

Printed in the USA
CPSIA information can be obtained
at www.ICGtesting.com
JSHW072028140824
68134JS00044B/3833